THE NEUFIT METHOD

THE
neufit
METHOD

Unleash the Power of the Nervous System
for Faster Healing and Optimal Performance

GARRETT SALPETER

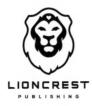

LIONCREST
PUBLISHING

THE NEUFIT METHOD
Unleash the Power of the Nervous System for
Faster Healing and Optimal Performance

ISBN   978-1-5445-2092-6 *Hardcover*
           978-1-5445-2091-9 *Paperback*
           978-1-5445-2090-2 *Ebook*

To Briana, for your support and partnership on this journey. To Gwenny, thank you for being our "Gwen-spiration." To Gemma, the "sparkly Gem" that lights up our lives.

And to Team NeuFit and all of the NeuFit practitioners around the world: thank you for your commitment to upgrading rehabilitation and fitness.

CONTENTS

DISCLAIMER 1

INTRODUCTION 3

1. OUR HIDDEN NEUROLOGICAL POTENTIAL 17

PART 1: THE NEUFIT METHOD FOR REHABILITATION

2. THE NEUFIT METHOD FOR RECOVERING FROM INJURY 37

3. THE NEUFIT METHOD FOR RECOVERING FROM SURGERY 51

4. THE NEUFIT METHOD FOR TREATING CHRONIC PAIN 65

5. THE NEUFIT METHOD FOR TREATING NEUROLOGICAL CONDITIONS ... 81

PART 2: THE NEUFIT METHOD FOR FITNESS TRAINING AND HIGH PERFORMANCE

6. THE NEUFIT METHOD FOR LONG-TERM FITNESS 105

7. THE NEUFIT METHOD FOR ELITE ATHLETIC PERFORMANCE 135

PART 3: THE NEUFIT METHOD FOR SUSTAINABLE NEUROLOGICAL HEALTH

8. HOW TO ASSESS NERVOUS SYSTEM HEALTH: THE PRIMARY INDICATORS.......... 173

9. THE NEUFIT METHOD FOR LIFELONG NEUROLOGICAL HEALTH........................ 205

CONCLUSION.. 247

APPENDIX 1... 255

APPENDIX 2... 259

ACKNOWLEDGMENTS... 267

ABOUT THE AUTHOR 271

REFERENCES 273

DISCLAIMER

This book contains a number of client stories. In some cases, we have permission to use clients' actual or full names. However, in some examples, we refer to clients on a first-name basis and/or have changed their names to protect their privacy. Either way, all of the client stories included in this book are accurate accounts of their experiences with NeuFit.

In addition to client stories, this book contains health-related advice and information, including concepts that NeuFit practitioners use. If you are not a medical professional, please note that the information in this book should be used to supplement rather than replace the advice of your doctor or another trained health professional. Please seek the guidance of a physician or other medical professional before attempting any medical treatment, training routine, or lifestyle modification.

We have made every effort to ensure the accuracy of the information contained in this book as of the date of publication. This publisher and author, however, cannot be responsible for how readers choose to use the information, and we disclaim liability for any medical outcomes that may occur as a result of applying the methods suggested in this book.

INTRODUCTION

Amy was thrown from a horse when she was twenty-one years old. After being rushed to the hospital, she learned that her neck was broken in two places, along with one of the vertebrae in her thoracic spine. She was paralyzed from the chest down.

For nearly a week, she was unable to breathe on her own. She spent thirty days in the hospital and another five months in a rehab facility.

After a year of outpatient therapy, Amy recovered some feeling and movement below her chest, but it wasn't enough to function. For the next twenty-five years, she experimented with multiple forms of rehab and physical therapy, doing everything she could to regain function and improve her quality of life.

"I sometimes made a little bit of progress," she said, "but not enough to make an actual difference." In the meantime, doctors and physical therapists continued to tell her she would never walk again.

When she came to NeuFit for an initial evaluation, Amy didn't know what to expect. "Let's just see what happens," she told herself.

We started her treatment with fifteen minutes of electrical stimulation therapy, targeting the pathways between her brain and nervous system. "That was on a Monday," Amy said. "Tuesday night when I went to sleep, I woke up at two o'clock in the morning and felt like I could move my leg."

After thinking it over for a few minutes, she decided to give it a try. To her amazement, for the first time in twenty-five years, Amy was able to pull her left leg toward her chest. "And that was after one session!"

How was this possible? And why had over two decades in rehab and physical therapy produced such disappointing results for her up to that point?

THE LIMITS OF A TRADITIONAL REHAB APPROACH

Traditional approaches to rehab often focus on the bones and tissues, or the equivalent of the body's hardware. When someone has a neurological injury like Amy's—or another type of injury or chronic pain—they often assume that treating the body's physical structure is the best way to fix the problem.

This is why people commonly turn to surgery, joint braces, anti-inflammatory medicines, and/or conventional physical therapy in an attempt to mend what's broken.

Though these approaches can alleviate the physical damage to the body, they often fail to address the underlying cause of that damage, not to mention the body's dysfunctional response to the original injury. As a result, conventional, hardware-focused treatments tend to have a limited impact on patients' long-term healing and health.

When their doctors and therapists focus exclusively on the body's physical structure, patients often struggle to fully recover and regain strength and range of motion. In the meantime, patients like Amy frequently hit a wall when it comes to improving their ability to function.

The limits of a conventional approach to rehab apply in a fitness training context as well. Even if someone is able to make the transition from rehab to training, traditional training methods typically focus on the body's physical structure. More often than not, these methods don't give the body the stimulation it needs to achieve meaningful results and perform at peak levels.

THE POWER IN THE BODY'S SOFTWARE

As Amy's experience demonstrates, we have the potential to make a major difference in both healing and performance without changing the body's physical structure—its hardware—at all. How? By reprogramming the brain and nervous system, or the equivalent of the body's software.

Like a computer's operating system, the brain and nervous system send signals that influence the way every part of the body runs and interacts.

In other words, the nervous system software controls the body's hardware, affecting how the bones, muscles, connective tissue, and organs function and work together. Since the nervous system impacts almost every function in the human body, focusing on the nervous system during rehab and training can create profound improvements in healing and performance.

Amy's experience shows how this works in practice. One NeuFit session definitely wasn't enough for her body to heal any of its structural hardware or repair her original spinal cord injury. Instead, it was a shift in her neurological software that helped her progress more quickly than she ever thought possible.

REWIRING THE BRAIN

Amy's story is one of many examples of the power of a nervous system-centered or neurological approach to rehab and fitness. How exactly does this approach work?

It starts with creating changes in the brain. As the body's command center, the brain controls the nervous system. Thanks to evolution, the brain is always more concerned with short-term survival than long-term performance. It's constantly working to protect us.

In its quest to protect us, though, the brain often blocks the body's innate potential. (We'll dig deeper into the brain's survival bias and the implications for rehab and performance in Chapter 1.)

Though most people have more strength and more range of motion than they realize, the brain and nervous system often inhibit these capabilities. Whether it's due to poor habits or responses to trauma, the brain tends to impose "governors" or limitations on the body in the interest of survival and protection.

These limitations can show up in a variety of ways. Sometimes, the brain creates tension in the body to keep it from moving or stretching too far. Sometimes, it sends a pain signal in an attempt to limit movement. Sometimes, it limits the speed of movement. Other times, it reduces muscle strength to the point where we decrease the load or avoid loading certain areas of the body altogether because the brain believes they're compromised—even if these areas are not actually compromised.

SHIFTING AMY'S NEUROLOGICAL PROGRAMMING

Amy's experience is a classic example of how the brain's survival bias can hold back the body's healing process. In order to protect her body, her brain was keeping her from expressing her ability to lift her leg toward her chest due to a phenomenon known as learned disuse (a concept we'll explore in more detail in the chapters that follow).

When she moved her leg after that first session, she was tapping into an existing reservoir of functional ability. Up to that point, her brain's survival programming had been blocking that ability, causing it to lie dormant.

By using electrical stimulation to create different neurological inputs, we effectively changed the software commands Amy's brain was sending to her nervous system. Through this process of neuromuscular re-education, her body learned to use its hardware more and more effectively over time.

GOING BEYOND THE LIMITS

After that initial treatment session, Amy started coming to NeuFit three times per week, and she kept making headway. In each session, we combined electrical stimulation therapy with movements designed to reconnect the pathways between her brain and nervous system. "It wasn't a sacrifice to put in the effort," she said, "because it was just amazing to see the results."

As time went by, she continued to experience meaningful neurological changes: "I can now feel hot and cold temperatures," she added. "And my sensation level overall has just gotten better." She also started to sweat below the area of her injury. What was the significance of these milestones? They were clear signs that her sensory and autonomic nervous systems were coming back on line, paving the way for motor recovery.

In the meantime, she regained strength and mobility. "All of my muscles have gotten stronger," she said. "When I first came in, my hamstrings did not work at all. I couldn't even try to contract them, let alone get any movement out of them." A year into working with NeuFit, she could not only engage her hamstrings but also use them to move her legs.

After two years of hard work, Amy was ready to show off her progress. She organized a party with a group of her relatives at a restaurant in Austin, arranging for them to arrive early so she could make her grand entrance. When she walked into the restaurant with a walker, her family burst into tears.

After twenty-five years of being paralyzed, they assumed Amy would have to spend the rest of her life in a wheelchair. They never imagined she would walk again.

TRANSFORMING REHAB AND PERFORMANCE

After witnessing so many stories like Amy's and seeing the extraordinary results of neurologically focused rehabilitation and training, it's easy to understand why thousands of practitioners and patients have embraced this approach.

Whether we want to address internal health or external performance, whether we're talking about the general population or elite athletes, our work at the neurological level has the potential to generate immediate *and* sustainable results.

In this book, we'll look at various ways electrical stimulation and neurological interventions support both healing and optimal performance. Again, since the nervous system controls and is intimately connected with every part of the body, taking a neurological approach to rehab and training can benefit a wide range of individuals, including:

- People suffering from injury
- People recovering from surgery
- People with chronic pain
- People with spinal cord injuries and neurological challenges or diseases
- People transitioning from rehab to training
- People looking to optimize fitness for health and longevity
- Athletes who want to reach and sustain an optimal level of performance

Besides sharing best practices for treating each of these populations by focusing on the brain and nervous system, this book also explores the advantages of electrical stimulation therapy for enhancing the body's natural processes of adaptation and growth.

The book also lays out the building blocks of an optimal neurologically focused treatment cycle, from rehab to training for long-term fitness and optimal health and performance. Finally, it offers specific, practical strategies for tapping into hidden neurological potential, achieving greater levels of neurological activation and control, accelerating healing and recovery, and performing better—inside and outside the therapy clinic or gym.

MY NEUROLOGICAL EPIPHANY

I've always had a passion for physiology. Growing up as a hockey player, I was constantly looking for ways to use physiology to become a better athlete. Though I didn't have the words for it at the time, I believed my body was adaptable and that I could train it to grow and compete at the highest levels. As long as I put in the work, I thought, there were no limits to what I could achieve on the ice.

I worked with some of the best trainers in my area, who had me do things like weight lifting, sprint intervals, and agility drills—all with the goal of helping me improve my performance. But I continued to get frustrated with the lack of results. Though their traditional approaches to training helped me get bigger and stronger, I couldn't translate those improvements into better performance or increased speed on the ice.

Besides hitting that speed wall, I also got injured during those years, tearing a labrum in my hip and developing a "stress fracture" in my lumbar spine (a spondylolisthesis). Naturally, I wanted to get back on the ice as quickly as possible, so I sought out several physical therapists, hoping they might help me. I also visited a few orthopedic surgeons to hear their opinions.

Their prescriptions were underwhelming. Some of them told me to use a back brace or take anti-inflammatory pills. Others prescribed more powerful drugs. Others recommended surgery. Others told me to rest. I felt both disappointed and powerless. And I became convinced that there had to be a better way to approach recovery and training.

Eventually, I recovered from my injuries, and I went on to play hockey in college. In the meantime, I decided to channel my enthusiasm for problem-solving into a physics and engineering degree.

A LUCKY INJURY?

Toward the end of my college hockey career, I tore a ligament in my wrist. The doctors recommended surgery, telling me I wouldn't be able to return to the ice for several months. Resigned to a traditional, hardware-based approach to injury treatment, I assumed surgery was my only option.

A few days before my scheduled surgery, I went to see a chiropractic neurologist. He took an approach to rehab I'd never seen before: using manual techniques that focused on changing the neurological responses to the damage, he stimulated the muscles around my wrist injury.

Then he introduced me to a machine that used direct electrical current to help stimulate tissue healing. After a single treatment, I was amazed at how much the pain diminished and at how much range of motion I regained. And I wanted to understand why.

By working neurologically, the doctor explained, he was putting the body in a state where it could heal the ligaments on its own. How? In part, it was by reprogramming the brain at a global level, helping it shift resources away from survival and protection—and toward regeneration and recovery. That global shift also had effects at the local level, increasing the flow of blood and nutrients to the injured tissue, as well as reactivating the relevant muscles to protect the injured area as it healed.

After a series of these neurologically focused treatments, I was able to avoid surgery. Not only that, but I was back on the ice in three weeks instead of three months, and I recovered full strength and movement in my wrist.

For the first time in my life as an athlete, the experience of rehab felt mind-blowing, not to mention empowering and invigorating. I observed first-hand how the combination of neurology and technology could help the body tap into its natural capacity to heal. Ultimately, I realized it was all about sending the right signals to and from the brain to the nervous system.

LAUNCHING A NEW TECHNOLOGY

After experiencing the power of the neurological approach and the effects of direct electrical current in my own recovery process, I was determined to share my experience with as many people as possible.

I went on to earn a master's degree in engineering, and I apprenticed with several doctors and therapists, including the chiropractic neurologist who first introduced me to neurological rehab techniques.

As I was completing my degree, I opened a new practice within a local doctor's office, applying the functional neurology protocols I'd learned from my mentors and from self-study of leading-edge neurological research.

As my practice grew, I continued to refine my treatment and training methods. I also spotted opportunities to improve the direct current technology we used. How could we increase the power without damaging the skin or eliciting a stress response in the body? How could we adjust the waveform, power, and frequency on the machine to fit all stages of rehabilitation and fitness training?

After waiting in vain for someone else to reinvent the technology, I finally decided to do it myself. In collaboration with a small group of electrical engineering colleagues, I created the Neubie, which stands for "Neuro-Bio-Electric" stimulator. It's a patented, FDA-cleared[1] device that uses direct electrical current to stimulate the nervous system. (Chapter 1 goes into more detail about how the Neubie works.)

I started out working with people similar to me: athletes who wanted to recover faster from injury and return to the playing field as quickly as possible. As word spread, the flagship NeuFit clinic began to attract people dealing with chronic pain, traumatic brain injuries, stroke, multiple sclerosis, and spinal cord injuries like Amy's.

Over the past several years, a growing number of physical therapy and chiropractic clinics, hospitals, nursing homes, fitness facilities, and integrative medicine practitioners across the country have started using the NeuFit Method and the Neubie for healing, recovery, and performance. I share some of their stories throughout the chapters of this book.

In addition, more and more athletes and sports teams at the high school, university, and professional levels are integrating NeuFit's treatment approach into their rehab programs.

As of this writing, the University of Texas, Ohio State University, Georgia Tech, the Chicago Cubs, the Washington Nationals, the Washington Football Team, the Boston Red Sox, the L.A. Angels, the L.A. Clippers, the L.A. Dodgers, the San José Sharks, the Pittsburgh Pirates, the Carolina Panthers, Austin FC, and the Columbus Crew have used or are using the NeuFit Method and the Neubie to improve recovery and performance.

THE IMPACT OF ELECTRICAL STIMULATION ON FITNESS AND PERFORMANCE

In the process of helping thousands of clients transition from rehab into training, I've discovered that direct electrical current can also have a significant positive impact on long-term fitness and performance.

Over and over, I've observed how the right kind of neurological stimulation helps athletes push well beyond their comfort zones, enhancing the benefits of exercise even as it minimizes their risk of injury (or re-injury).

As it turns out, the same neurological principles that are so effective for recovery also provide a tremendous boost to training. By enhancing muscle recruitment, or helping people use more of their existing muscle, neurological stimulation gives them virtually all the benefits of heavy lifting and resistance training without having to lift nearly as much weight—or risk the associated strain on the body's joints.

When it comes to fitness and performance, the benefits of a neurological approach aren't limited to elite athletes. Working neurologically can also have a profound impact on anyone who cares about their health and wants to perform at their highest level, no matter their age or athletic ability.

HOW TO USE THIS BOOK

After explaining the foundational neurological principles at the core of the NeuFit Method, Part 1 of this book lays out the essentials of a neurological approach to rehab. It also looks at the advantages of a functional (nervous system) versus a structural (bone and tissue) approach to recovery in the context of injury rehab, post-surgical rehab, chronic pain, and neurological injuries or diseases.

Through specific examples, the chapters in Part 1 illustrate how working at the level of the brain and nervous system can optimize and accelerate the healing process—and help prevent re-injury and/or loss of function in the long-term.

In Part 2, the focus is on the transition from rehab to training and on how to build a bridge from recovery to long-term fitness and high performance. Part 2 also looks at the ways the brain sacrifices long-term performance for short-term survival—and explores how to change neurological programming to achieve optimal performance for both the general population and elite athletes.

Part 3 dives more deeply into nervous system health. It

lays out the most important indicators of nervous system function, including heart rate variability, sleep quality, digestion, immune function, and energy level. It also explains how to interpret these indicators to optimize recovery and performance.

Besides guiding rehabilitation and training, the indicators of nervous system function show how our lifestyle choices affect our neurological health. With this in mind, Part 3 also offers practical lifestyle strategies to improve and sustain neurological health for the long haul. In addition to sharing best practices for nervous system-strengthening nutrition, sleep hygiene, and general movement, it integrates breathing practices designed to dramatically improve nervous system function.

Though it incorporates plenty of research to demonstrate the benefits of a neurological approach to rehab and training, this book is not an academic treatise on the value of nervous-system-focused physical therapy. Nor is it an advertisement for using electrical stimulation in recovery and training.

With this book, my goal is to share the power and potential of a neurology-first approach to rehab and long-term fitness. I've designed it to help both practitioners and patients learn how to tap into their hidden neurological potential and break through their self-imposed limitations.

What happens when we remove the obstacles to healing and high performance? What's possible when we unleash the body's full capacity to adapt and grow? The answers are in the pages that follow.

1

OUR HIDDEN NEUROLOGICAL POTENTIAL

By the time he stumbled into the NeuFit clinic, Rob's back hurt so badly he could hardly move. Even after multiple doses of opioid pain medication, he rated his pain a ten on a scale of one to ten.

As a computer scientist, Rob spent long days at the office, where he sat down most of the time. He played pick-up soccer a few times a week, but he wasn't very active otherwise. From time to time, he felt some discomfort in his back—a bit of stiffness here, some minor pain there—but it never amounted to anything serious.

One day at work, he bent down to pick up a pen he'd dropped on the floor. Suddenly, seemingly out of nowhere, his back seized up. He sank to the floor, doubled over in pain.

He made an emergency visit to his doctor, who prescribed bed rest and painkillers. Neither gave him any relief. For the next three days, he limped between his bed and the bathroom, doing his best to keep his spine immobilized. Every movement, no matter how minor, was agonizing.

As soon as he made it to our treatment table, we hooked up Rob to the Neubie. He was as skeptical as he was desperate. "I doubt you can help me," he said, wincing, "but I'm willing to try anything."

First, we did a body scan, searching for the places where his nervous system was triggering the spasms that were compounding his pain.

Then we placed the electricity-conducting pads in the spots where his body's reaction to the machine was most intense, which weren't the same places he was feeling the pain (Why? We'll explore this phenomenon in more depth later in this chapter, as well as in Chapter 4).

As we stimulated his muscles with electrical current, we asked him to do a series of subtle movements to engage the muscles, starting with reaching his feet toward the corners of the table one inch at a time.

"I can't move any more than that!" he said. But he didn't need to: alternating those movements of his feet created a mild rocking movement in his pelvis, which created a gentle rotation in the lower back.

As the minutes passed, his range of motion increased inch by inch. After ten minutes, he was able to roll over onto his hands and knees. "I can't believe this!" he said, sighing with relief, "I thought I was going to be a hunchback from now on."

WHY DOES THE BODY OVERREACT?

Had he actually "thrown out" his back, Rob would have landed in the emergency room and immediately gone into surgery. He might have even been paralyzed.

In reality, though, the issue was not in the structure, or hardware, of his body. How did we know? His quick response to neurologically focused treatment and stimulation with the Neubie was proof.

In Rob's case, and in so many cases like his, the problem was at the level of the nervous system—what we at NeuFit refer to as the body's software. There was likely some pressure or irritation on a nerve root exiting his spinal cord (which is common in situations where people "throw out" their backs). In response to that irritation, Rob's brain sounded an alarm, sending a pain signal and causing major muscle spasms to protect the area against further damage.

Why did Rob's body respond this way? And why does the body tend to "overreact" in situations like his?

Over time, whether it's due to poor habits or responses to bodily trauma, the brain tends to impose governors, or limiting signals, on the body. As I wrote in the introduction, these governors can physically manifest in a variety of ways. Sometimes, they shut down the body, inhibiting certain muscles in order to weaken them. Other times, they keep certain areas of the body tight or stiff. Sometimes, as Rob experienced, they send a pain signal and lock down the body with spasms in an attempt to restrict movement.

Why does this happen? What are the consequences? And how

can we change the brain's software to reprogram neurological signals that limit the body?

THE BRAIN IS HARDWIRED FOR SURVIVAL AND PROTECTION

As I mentioned in the introduction, the brain limits the body in order to protect it and help it survive. Its default programming, which has evolved over tens of thousands of years, is to constantly scan the environment, looking for signs of danger and threats to safety.

Look at this picture of the spectators at a Major League Baseball game (Figure 1-1). Do you notice anything in particular about how they react to the foul ball flying toward them?

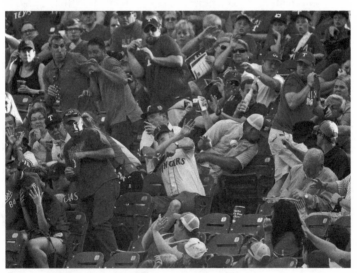

Figure 1-1: Spectators at a baseball game react to a foul ball.
Source: Getty Images

As soon as the ball leaves the player's bat and flies into the stands, all the spectators instantly raise their arms, demonstrating the same hardwired reflex to protect their faces. Their reaction is just one example of how humans naturally respond to the brain's desire to keep us safe.

When a baseball is hurtling toward us, we react immediately, without thinking. We bring the hard, bony parts of our body in front of the softer, more vulnerable areas like the eyes and the internal organs. In that moment, our survival takes priority over everything else. We forget about the conversation we were having. We drop our beer.

Any time we're in a situation where the brain perceives something that's an immediate threat to survival, everything else becomes secondary—including healing and performance.

MISREADING THREATS TO SURVIVAL

Obviously, the brain's protective reflex is helpful in scenarios where there's a genuine threat to survival, such as when a baseball is flying toward us.

However, there are many times when a situation doesn't warrant a reaction that might have been appropriate ten thousand years ago when we were fleeing predators or enemies. In other words, the brain's response doesn't always match the circumstances, and the brain often misinterprets or overestimates the actual level of threat.

In light of the fact that the brain processes approximately ten to twenty million bits of information every second, this is no surprise.[2]

As it sorts through all of this information, the brain is constantly searching for danger signs. Given the astounding amount of data it's processing, it's understandable that the brain sometimes misjudges the level of threat. However, this misjudgment has consequences. Every time the brain senses danger, it sends signals to the nervous system that produce a stress response in the body—and limit the body in some way.

THE EFFECTS OF THE BRAIN'S SURVIVAL BIAS

The brain's natural tendency to prioritize survival and protection can have both immediate and long-term consequences for rehab, performance, and the ability to function on a day-to-day basis.

In Rob's case, for example, his brain perceived that he was moving in a way that was threatening. In response, his brain sent a signal to the nervous system to do whatever it took to protect his back, basically immobilizing him.

Besides triggering things like muscle spasms, the brain's survival bias also impacts the body's response to trauma—and often inhibits the body's potential to heal itself. If someone has a tear in the pec muscle or the hamstring muscle, for example, the body takes its cues from the brain, bracing and guarding around the area of injury as if it's preparing for an attack.

Though this physiological response makes sense in light of the brain's default programming, it's very counterproductive for healing. Why? All of the tension around the area of injury reduces muscle movement, which in turn diminishes the flow of blood and nutrients necessary for recovery.[3] As a result, the body can take weeks, or even months, to bounce back from even minor injuries because it can't channel energy and resources where they're needed most.

What happens in the body after surgery, particularly after orthopedic surgery, is similar. When someone has knee or shoulder surgery, for example, the body usually doesn't understand that it's been through a process of repair. Since the brain perceives surgery as trauma and an acute threat to survival, the body reacts to the operation as if it's been invaded, stabbed, torn up.

Immediately after surgery, the brain basically orders the body to stiffen some muscles and inhibit (or "deactivate") others to protect itself from further damage. This deactivation is what leads to the muscle atrophy that follows most surgeries, which can happen surprisingly quickly.

Because of these responses to surgery, it sometimes takes years for the body to fully recover from an operation. In fact, the body's *response* to the trauma of surgery is often worse and more harmful over time than the trauma that led to the operation in the first place.

The brain's natural tendency to prioritize survival and protection over healing and long-term performance also may have major implications for people dealing with chronic pain and neurological injuries or diseases.

Why was Amy (from the introduction), who was paralyzed from the chest down at age twenty-one, unable to lift her leg to her chest for twenty-five years? At some point after her accident, she'd actually regained the ability to lift her leg. But her brain had learned to avoid that movement. It was intentionally limiting that output and suppressing her capacity to move in order to protect her body.

The bottom line is this: when left to its own devices, the brain

almost always sacrifices long-term health for short-term survival.
In terms of athletic performance, this neurological tendency
can have a huge impact on factors like range of motion, speed,
strength, and resilience.

The fact is that the brain cares more about ensuring we live
to see tomorrow than helping improve performance. Things
like increasing the speed of our fastball by five miles per hour,
raising our vertical jump by a few inches, or shaving a few
seconds off our mile time automatically take a back seat to
immediate threats.

As a result, even among athletes competing at the highest
levels, the brain's natural inclination is to actively inhibit the
body. It will do everything in its power to keep us from moving
too far or too fast or exerting too much force and getting
injured. According to the brain's ten-thousand-year-old programming, getting injured means we're less likely to outrun
predators—and more likely to get eaten.

HOW THE BRAIN'S SURVIVAL BIAS
AFFECTS COGNITIVE FUNCTION

Besides physical function, the brain's natural tendency to prioritize
survival over everything else can also affect cognitive function.

Why does this happen? Physiologically speaking, the brain will always
"feed" its lower, survival-oriented areas first. So if your energy levels
are low, the brain won't have enough fuel to supply the higher, more
recently evolved areas that perform executive functions. In other
words, as the energy level in the frontal lobe of the brain gets diminished, so does the capacity for clear thinking and problem-solving.

Imagine, for example, that the "higher" and "lower" parts of the brain both need seventy units of energy, or 140 total units of energy. But let's say the body only has access to 100 units of energy.

In this scenario, the parts of the brain dedicated to survival will automatically take seventy of those 100 units of energy since their needs prevail over those in the higher centers of the brain. As a result, the more evolved parts of the brain get the short end of the stick, ending up with only thirty of those units of energy—which isn't enough to fuel optimal executive function. This leads to poor decision-making and impaired intellectual ability, which can affect everything from performance on an academic test to making unhealthy food choices to losing your temper with colleagues or family members.

THE GOOD NEWS: NEUROPLASTICITY AND THE BRAIN'S CAPACITY TO CHANGE

Though the brain is automatically programmed for survival and protection, here's the good news: it's entirely possible to change or upgrade that programming. This is due to a phenomenon known as neuroplasticity.

Neuroplasticity is a concept that describes the ability of the brain and the nervous system to change and adapt over time. Depending on the nature of the neurological inputs, these changes and adaptations can go in either a positive or negative direction. This is called specificity of adaptation, which Chapter 5 covers in more detail.

For now, it's important to focus on the fact that it's possible to affect both the direction and the magnitude of neuroplasticity to a much greater degree than previously thought.

In the past, scientists and medical experts assumed the brain and nervous system were hardwired. After childhood, they thought there was little room for neurological improvement or development.

However, over the past two decades, researchers have continued to learn more about the true nature of neuroplasticity. Their findings are as startling as they are encouraging.

As it turns out, we have the potential to affect the brain and nervous system over the entire course of a person's life—not just in childhood. For people recovering from injury or surgery, the potential for neuroplastic change presents an opportunity for faster healing.[4]

For people dealing with chronic pain or neurological conditions, neuroplasticity can increase the chances of restoring movement and function. For athletes and others looking to optimize fitness and performance, the nature of neuroplasticity means they have the ability to train and compete at levels beyond what they previously thought possible.

HARNESSING THE POTENTIAL OF NEUROPLASTICITY

Given the nature of neuroplasticity, what factors cause positive neuroplastic changes versus negative ones? How can we capitalize on the innate potential of neuroplasticity to support healing and improve performance? And how can we utilize neuroplasticity to enhance brain and nervous system function—and overall quality of life—in the long term?

When it comes to creating positive neuroplastic changes,

there are two major prerequisites: physiological support and neurological stimulation.

Just as you need resilient materials like bricks and concrete to lay the groundwork for a house, the body needs a healthy, vibrant, and robust physiological foundation for positive neuroplastic changes to happen.

Obviously, nutrition plays a key role here: not only does the body rely on specific proteins to build nerves and nervous system tissues, but it also needs energy from high-quality fats, along with some carbohydrates, to support brain and nervous system function.

In addition to nutrition, reducing or controlling inflammation is another necessary ingredient in healthy neuroplastic adaptations. Sleep is also a significant factor since building and upgrading neural pathways happens during sleep. Chapter 9 outlines specific strategies for nervous system-centered nutrition, sleep, and other lifestyle factors that help reinforce positive neuroplastic development.

In the meantime, let's take a closer look at the other crucial requirement for productive neuroplastic change: neurological stimulation. Just as consistent training at the gym helps strengthen the muscles, consistent neurological stimulation can strengthen the nervous system by supporting the development of new neurological pathways, improving the function of existing pathways, and even repairing damaged ones.

If we don't exercise, the body tends to grow weaker, more rigid, and/or more easily fatigued. Similarly, our capacity to recover or strengthen brain and nervous system function diminishes in the absence of neurological stimulation—or in the absence of *the right kind* of neurological stimulation.

This is the dark side of neuroplasticity, which is known as learned disuse, a concept we'll examine in more detail in Chapter 5. Meanwhile, let's take a closer look at what the right kind of neurological stimulation looks like.

THE OPTIMAL APPROACH TO NEUROLOGICAL STIMULATION

If neurological stimulation is one of the keys to positive neuroplastic changes, what's the best way to approach it? There are three important criteria:

1. It needs to be consistent.
2. It needs to have a sufficient level of intensity.
3. It needs to be strategic and specifically targeted to nerve pathways that show deficits and have the potential for repair and growth.

Neurological stimulation that combines all three of these criteria can generate lasting positive neuroplastic changes in the brain and nervous system.

At the same time, it's important to keep in mind that it can take an enormous amount of time and effort to create positive neuroplastic changes. Several recent studies of people recovering from a stroke,[5] for example, suggest that the amount of work patients perform in a standard therapy session is far too little to generate meaningful neuroplastic changes.

According to the latest research, creating significant neuroplastic change and restoring function requires *hundreds of thousands* of repetitions of various movements and tasks. This translates into hundreds or thousands of repetitions in *each* therapy session, which can end up feeling more like a training session for a professional athlete than a typical physical therapy treatment.

When it comes to making meaningful neuroplastic changes, stroke or spinal cord injury patients aren't the only ones who need to invest significant time and effort. Whether someone is recovering from injury or surgery, suffering from chronic pain, or training for long-term health and elite performance, there's still significant work involved in driving neuroplasticity—and ensuring that neuroplastic changes head in a positive direction.

ENTER THE NEUBIE

As I mentioned in the introduction, I was inspired to share the healing potential of the neurological approach to treatment after I experienced its effects first-hand. But even as I continued to witness the therapeutic impacts of the neurology-first approach—and learn more about electrical current's power to re-educate the nervous system—I realized there was a missing piece.

As an engineer, it was clear to me that there was a way to improve on the direct current technology we were using to further accelerate healing and help people move past their bodies' self-imposed limitations. In other words, I knew it was possible to create a device that could harness a more powerful, more precise direct current signal that was both safe and effective.

When I realized no one else was going to develop the machine I envisioned, I decided to build it myself. In 2017, after years of trial and error, not to mention hundreds of safety tests, my team and I officially introduced the Neubie (which stands for **Neu**ro-**Bio**-Electric Stimulator), a patented device that uses direct electrical current to stimulate the brain and nervous system and re-educate the muscles for recovery and growth.

WHAT SETS THE NEUBIE APART?

Unlike traditional electrical stimulation devices, the Neubie is able to harness the benefits of direct current on tissue healing and re-educate the nervous system to improve its function. Since it uses a special carrier waveform, the Neubie does this without damaging the skin or producing a stress response in the body (as direct current devices typically did in the past, which is why they never became widely used).

Even though direct current (DC) has proven positive effects on tissue healing and nervous system function,[6] virtually every electrical stimulation machine available today uses alternating current (AC).

Though there are some benefits at lower levels of alternating current, the effects can be problematic at higher therapeutic levels. Instead of teaching the muscles to work together more efficiently, alternating current often trains them to grow more rigid over time.

When turned up to a level high enough to impact neuromuscular function, alternating current actually causes the muscles to fight against one other, or co-contract, locking up the body so it's unable to move.

In contrast, the Neubie can have a different effect both because its waveform is designed to match the rate at which electrical charges transfer across nerves and because it uses direct current, which is what the nervous system uses.

That is, the pathways of the nervous system send signals in one direction and in one direction only. They're similar to a highway, where there's a set of lanes in which traffic moves in one direction and a separate set of lanes in which cars travel in the opposite direction.

In the nervous system, one pathway conducts impulses from the brain to the body, issuing motor commands from the brain, instructing the body to take some sort of action. Meanwhile, separate sensory pathways in the nervous system carry signals from the body to the brain. In other words, the same nervous system pathways that conduct signals from the brain to the body will never transmit signals in the other direction, from the body to the brain.

Since it closely resembles the nervous system's natural way of operating, the Neubie's use of direct current synchronizes as much as possible with the human body.

In this way, the stimulation signals from the Neubie minimize the protective responses and muscular co-contractions that would otherwise increase resistance in the body. With less co-contraction, it's easier for the input signal to stimulate the sensory pathways. This enhanced neurological input creates a foundation for a powerful form of muscular re-education. At the same time, the Neubie helps increase parasympathetic (rest and digest) nervous system activity, which activates the body's inherent capacity to heal and perform at an optimal level.

HOW THE NEUBIE TRANSFORMED A
PHYSICAL THERAPY PRACTICE

At most physical therapy practices, the owner is the one patients always want to see, since the owner is the one with the most knowledge and experience. But once I taught all my other therapists how to use the Neubie, patients are excited to go to any therapist on our staff.

With the Neubie as part of our treatment process, we're able to pinpoint patients' trouble spots with 100 percent accuracy. We tell patients they can expect to have some sort of positive outcome within four sessions. Every therapist in my practice is trained to use the machine and can produce these results.

I brought the Neubie into my practice in January 2018. I quickly went from one Neubie to three. By the end of 2018, my practice had 94 percent more revenue than in any previous year.

When they see how successful I've become, other clinicians ask me about my marketing plan. I tell them the biggest key is to find a practice differentiator. I've been a physical therapist for twenty-five years, and I've never found a practice differentiator like the Neubie.

—JASON WAZ, PHYSICAL THERAPIST AND FOUNDER OF COMPETITIVE EDGE PHYSICAL THERAPY IN TAMPA, FLORIDA

ACCELERATING HEALING BY ENHANCING THE BODY'S NATURAL PROCESSES

As powerful as the technology is, it's important to keep in mind that the Neubie isn't a replacement for the body's natural healing and repair processes. Instead, the device is designed to access the body's existing capacity—and raise it. Once the machine kick-starts the body's internal power sources, biological processes take over and do the rest.

As I mentioned at the beginning of this chapter, due to the brain's natural tendency to prioritize survival and protection, the body often limits itself when it comes to healing and performance. The Neubie's capacity for neuromuscular re-education changes that default neurological programming, upgrading the brain's software and helping the body's hardware function at a higher level over time.

Since the NeuFit Method (including the use of the Neubie) combines all the necessary components of effective neurological stimulation, it can dramatically speed up the healing process in cases of injury, as Rob's experience illustrates.

In Rob's case, as in all the injury-related cases we treat, we used a series of strategic neurological activation movements, combined with electrical stimulation from the Neubie, to relieve the pain in his back. Simply put, we sent signals to his brain that allowed it to register the edge of its current safety zone. By helping his brain determine that his body wasn't in danger, he was able to tone down the protective mechanisms of inhibition, tension, and pain.

The result? In just over twenty minutes, his pain decreased from a ten to a two. He went from hobbling into the clinic, hunched over in agony, to rolling onto his hands and knees, to standing up and jogging out the door.

Of course, all injuries are not created equal. Not everyone responds to the Neubie and the neurological approach to treatment as quickly or intensely as Rob did.

However, as we'll see in the chapters in Part 1, working neurologically to change the limiting patterns in the brain has the potential to reduce a person's pain and improve their quality of movement far more quickly—and far more effectively—than traditional approaches to rehab.

PART 1

THE NEUFIT METHOD FOR REHABILITATION

2

THE NEUFIT METHOD FOR RECOVERING FROM INJURY

As a football player at a major university in the Big 12 Conference, Randy was used to pushing himself to the maximum as much at practice as he did in games.

As a starting linebacker, he was also used to getting hurt. "A bruise here, a sore muscle there," he said. "It's just part of the game." Until his sophomore season, he'd never had an injury that kept him from missing more than a game or two.

One day at a mid-season practice, he went in for a hard tackle—and missed. He fell hard on the grass, landing directly on his right shoulder.

"I felt something shift," he said, "but I tried to shake it off." He quickly got to his feet. Then he tried to lift his arm: "It just felt frozen. Then when I tried to lift it, the pain was so sharp I thought I might pass out."

After a physical exam and an x-ray, the team doctor diagnosed him with a grade 2 separation of the acromioclavicular (A.C.) joint. In other words, he'd torn one of the ligaments that connected his collarbone to his shoulder blade.

"I didn't need surgery—that was the good news," Randy said. "The bad news was that it was going to take four to six weeks to heal."

For Randy, that meant sitting out the rest of the season. "I was so used to my body bouncing back from getting hurt," he said. "And I assumed this time would be no different. Getting that news was tough."

A NEUROLOGICAL INTERVENTION

About a week after Randy injured his shoulder, the university's athletic trainers invited the NeuFit team to their rehab facility. After hearing about other athletes' experiences with the neurological approach to rehab, they wanted to see how their players, including Randy, might respond to our treatment.

In Randy's case, we started off with a series of muscle tests, trying to gauge the state of the muscles in and around Randy's shoulder. Despite his best efforts, he could still only lift his arm about thirty degrees from his side.

We first used a few manual muscle activation techniques, stimulating various reflex points in his upper body.

Then we hooked Randy up to the Neubie. We performed a body scan, moving the electricity-conducting pads along different muscles and areas of his body, starting at a low power level and monitoring his response throughout.

His pain levels hovered between two and four out of ten. But when we got to his supraspinatus (the uppermost rotator cuff muscle) and teres minor (the lowest rotator cuff muscle), it was a different story. "Whoa!" he winced. "That's the spot right there." His pain level shot up from a four to an eight.

Once we zeroed in on those areas, we placed the pads on those spots and asked Randy to do some simple movements while we stimulated the muscles with the Neubie. First, we had him do a few circles with his shoulder blade. Then we asked him to raise his arm.

After a few minutes, he was able to lift his arm another twenty degrees. Another minute went by. His arm went up another thirty degrees. Before long, he raised his arm straight above his head. "I couldn't believe it," he said. "Fifteen minutes of treatment and I had full range of motion in my shoulder again!"

THE ORIGINAL TRAUMA AND THE BODY'S RESPONSE

As the example with Randy demonstrates, when someone is recovering from an injury, the biggest problem isn't necessarily the original trauma. Instead, as I mentioned in Chapter 1, the biggest barrier to healing is often *the body's response* to that trauma.

After he hurt his shoulder, Randy's brain and nervous system automatically sent signals to guard, protect, and brace around the area of injury. The pain he felt when he tried to raise his arm was actually an output signal from his brain.

Because his brain perceived that movement as a threat, it sent a pain signal to his arm. In other words, the brain's natural bias toward protection and survival was restricting Randy's movements, keeping him firmly inside his comfort zone to minimize the risk of making the injury worse.

However, all of these protective reactions can have serious downsides when it comes to recovering from injury. As we discussed in Chapter 1, excess tension inhibits the flow of blood and nutrients, which diminishes the body's ability to rebuild. On top of that, as the brain limits movement and signals muscles to shut down in certain areas, these compensatory movement patterns can make those areas of the body even more vulnerable to injury or re-injury.[7]

By addressing his injury at the level of the nervous system, we were able to identify exactly where Randy's neurological barriers were presenting themselves—and break through them.

Using electrical stimulation for neuromuscular re-education, we effectively changed the software commands his brain was sending to the nervous system, allowing his body to release its grip on the muscles and open the way for movement.

INJURY REHAB: THE NEUFIT METHOD

When the brain tries to protect the body after an original injury, it ends up creating governors, or limiting patterns, that restrict output and result in painful and/or limited movement. These governors also keep people from being able to fully rehabilitate and heal.

Based on my experience at NeuFit, I've concluded that managing these neurological responses is often the biggest factor in optimizing recovery from most injuries.

This is why we use a thorough three-step procedure at NeuFit that involves precisely identifying where the brain is imposing these neurological responses on the body, resetting those governors, and breaking through these self-imposed limitations to optimize the healing process.

Here's how the three-step procedure works:

Step 1: Identify. We start with a body mapping process to determine exactly where the nervous system is imposing governors or limitations on the body and restrictions in movement. This mapping process includes manual muscle testing as well as a body scan with the Neubie, where we move the electricity-conducting pads along the nerve pathways (as shown in Figure 2-1), searching for areas where the nervous system is limiting movement and muscle function. When we find these areas, the brain and nervous system usually try to protect against the signal, and it can feel especially intense for the patient, similar to a trigger point.

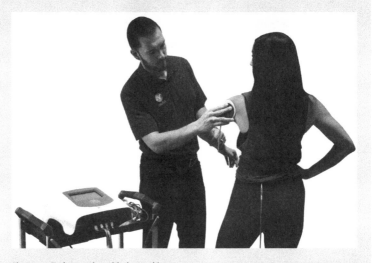

Figure 2-1: Body-mapping with the Neubie.

Step 2: Reset. Once we identify the areas where the body is imposing limiting patterns, we go about resetting those areas to change those patterns. Using manual muscle activation techniques and targeted electrical stimulation, combined with movements and exercises, we help change these neurological patterns and restore them to more normal, optimal function. Though some self-protection is necessary, these particular governors represent an overreaction in the body. By resetting or recalibrating the nervous system, we don't eliminate the self-protection reflex. Instead, we adjust it to the appropriate level.

Step 3: Breakthrough. Restoring function to muscles and tissues breaks through the obstacles that typically delay the healing process and opens up the recovery pathways for the body to heal more effectively. In the process, we also help patients access the range of motion, strength, and capacity for pain-free movement that's present but dormant—until we undo the limiting neurological patterns.

FUNCTION VERSUS STRUCTURE, SOFTWARE VERSUS HARDWARE

With acute or traumatic injuries, the neurological approach to rehab can significantly accelerate recovery times and decrease the risk of re-injury. At the same time, when we're weighing the best strategy for recovery, it's important to distinguish between the functional (software) and structural (hardware) aspects of an injury.

Randy's shoulder separation and Rob's back pain (as described in Chapter 1) are examples of injuries with a significant functional component. In both cases, the pain and limitations had more to do with changes at the muscular and nervous system level than with the initial injury or trauma.

With injuries like these, we can use direct electrical current to re-educate the body and shift the brain's software commands from survival and protection to healing and movement. Once this shift happens, the results are often immediate.

With injuries that have more of a structural/hardware component—i.e., injuries to the bones, joints, ligaments, and tissues—the rehab process is similar. The main difference is that recovery times are usually longer, depending on the nature and extent of the damage that needs to be repaired.

Even though structural injuries can take longer to heal, we can still increase both the speed and effectiveness of recovery by taking a neurological approach. Why? Addressing functional limitations removes the impediments that slow healing, and activating the right muscles helps support injured tissues as they heal, as Whitney's experience shows.

FROM A TORN ROTATOR CUFF TO MISS FITNESS OLYMPIA

Six weeks before IFBB (International Federation of Bodybuilding and Fitness) Pro Whitney Jones was set to defend her title at the 2019 Miss Fitness Olympia competition, she tore the labrum and a rotator cuff tendon in her left shoulder.

"They were pretty significant injuries, especially for my division," she said. "I didn't know what to do. I was six weeks out from the biggest show of the year, and I couldn't move my arm. It was literally just stuck to my side."

After getting her MRI results, which confirmed her injury, she started training with NeuFit. Though she'd heard of the technology, she'd never experienced it first-hand. "I never thought it would be as beneficial as it was. Within ten minutes, I was doing lateral raises with ten-pound dumbbells with no pain. I was a believer from that day on."

"In the lead up to the competition, I was getting treatments with NeuFit three times a week, in between routine training," she added. After practicing her competition routine for hours, it was nearly impossible to move her shoulder. "Then I would go in for treatment and get range of motion back. It also helped keep the muscles full so that I had the physique I needed to present on the Olympia stage."

For Whitney, NeuFit "was a crucial part of my prep and the success of my prep. If I had not been utilizing NeuFit, there was no way I would've made it to the stage, much less become two-time Miss Fitness Olympia."

RESTORING FUNCTION HELPS RESTORE STRUCTURE

How was Whitney able to bounce back from her shoulder injury so quickly—and go on to win Miss Fitness Olympia? Though there was a structural component to her injury, and though her body's hardware needed time to heal, working at the level of the brain and nervous system removed the barriers to that healing process.

Using electrical stimulation and muscle-activating exercises to reprogram the brain effectively changed her neurological software, allowing her body to direct resources and energy toward restoring its damaged hardware.

As Whitney's experience demonstrates, even when someone is dealing with a hardware injury that takes time to heal, restoring the body's functional capacity through neurological stimulation supports the structural healing process—and can significantly shorten recovery times.

With traditional approaches to rehab, recovery times for certain structural injuries are fairly fixed, though again, they tend to vary depending on the severity of the injury. For example, a torn rotator cuff like Whitney's typically takes four to six months to recover, depending on the size of the tear. A grade 2 shoulder separation like Randy's usually takes four to six weeks.

However, it's helpful to keep in mind that these assumptions around recovery times are based on conventional treatment methods that don't adequately address functional limitations, along with a healing process that's hindered by the brain's survival bias—and the associated limitations that survival bias imposes on the body.

Over the course of treating thousands of injuries, our experience at NeuFit is that working neurologically can upend traditional assumptions about recovery times—even with structural injuries. As of this writing, we have several injury treatment studies in the data collection phase, and we will share the results as they become available.

HOW THE NEUFIT METHOD AND THE NEUBIE TRANSFORMED A CHIROPRACTOR'S PRACTICE

The evolution and revolution in our practice have been incredible since we purchased the Neubie, with the patients we've used it on, with the results we've seen. It's changed the way we do things in our practice for the better.

A lot of difficult cases, things that would otherwise take months to materialize into positive outcomes, have gone down to weeks, including

*things like adhesive capsule issues, chronic low back pain, and radicular
back pain.*

*In my own case, I had a procedure in the summer, and I was back at
work within a month (of using the Neubie) after being told it would
take six to eight weeks, so the testimonial is personal as well.*

*On top of that, the Neubie was easy to incorporate naturally into
our existing practice because we were already working on a neuro-
functional model. We've rekindled the excitement in the clinic: not
only did the Neubie create a stir with patients, but it also created a
stir within our own staff. Everyone wants to experience it. The proof
is in the pudding with the product—and the results.*

—DR. ERNIE BAGNULO, CHIROPRACTOR, WIN HEALTH
SOLUTIONS, NIAGARA FALLS, ONTARIO, CANADA

TO REST, OR NOT TO REST?

A big part of injury rehab involves rebuilding the body's damaged structures and reinforcing them so they're more capable
of handling future challenges.

In the past, traditional approaches to injury rehab emphasized
the importance of rest in this rebuilding process. However,
even the strongest advocates of the rest, ice, compress, elevate (RICE) paradigm are starting to change their opinions,
including Dr. Gabe Mirkin.

Dr. Mirkin, who initially popularized the RICE methodology
in his best-selling *Sports Medicine Book* in 1978, recently shifted
his thinking around this approach. "Complete rest may delay
healing instead of helping," he wrote in 2015.[8]

Due to the neurological phenomenon known as specificity of adaptation (which we'll cover in detail in Chapter 5), the body adapts to get better at exactly what it's doing. When someone spends most of their time resting and being sedentary, the brain looks for ways to downregulate the systems of the body, including the delivery of nutrients to injured areas.

Unfortunately, this downregulation can have a negative impact on recovery, both in the short-term and the long-term. Why? Muscles, bones, and connective tissues need mechanical stimulus in order to regenerate. And just one day of unloading can begin to cause muscle atrophy.[9]

In addition to slowing the rate of healing, inactivity can also diminish the overall healing outcome. Take the example of the body repairing a muscle tear. Though the body will still find a way to heal if we don't move or load an injured muscle, the quality of the healed tissue will be less than optimal. As it tries to repair the damaged area, the body will lay down scar tissue in a random patchwork. Over time, this scar tissue can limit range of motion and cause muscles to weaken.[10]

By contrast, providing some level of load or mechanical force to injured muscle tissue (at a safe level, of course) helps regenerative cells orient themselves along the lines of force. In the process, instead of creating a random patchwork of scar tissue that ultimately limits movement, the body builds up high-quality tissue that enhances strength and range of motion in the area of injury. Along the way, it also minimizes the likelihood of re-injury.

Instead of allowing the muscles to lie dormant after injury, the neurological approach to injury rehab uses movement and stimulation—not rest—to facilitate recovery. In other words, safely and strategically stimulating the muscles doesn't just accelerate the healing process; it also steers it in the best possible direction.

ENSURING FULL RECOVERY AFTER INJURY

As exciting as it is to help people speed up the healing process after injury, it's also crucial to help them reach full recovery. With this goal in mind, we want to continuously evaluate their function and assess whether they might be creating compensatory patterns that could limit function and long-term performance.

When it comes to injury rehab, the ultimate goal is for patients to use the damaged part(s) of the body as if they hadn't experienced any trauma at all. From a neurological perspective, a patient hasn't completely recovered from an injury until they've regained full sensation and function in that area of the body.

Unfortunately, the completion of the recovery process is something that often gets overlooked in the world of rehab. So how do we know when recovery is complete? When we observe that the patient's strength, pain-free range of motion, movement velocity, and coordination—plus the function of all sensory receptors—are all back to optimal, pre-injury (or better) levels.

Let's return to the example of Randy, who separated his shoulder at football practice and regained full range of motion after fifteen minutes of neurological stimulation therapy.

After he recovered his range of motion, we asked him to try a pushup on his knees. "At that point, I didn't feel any pain," he said. "So I went from my knees to my feet and did ten more. And I still didn't feel any pain."

Later that day, his trainers continued to increase the level of challenge in another workout while monitoring his responses and assessing his neuromuscular capacity. After taking him through multiple rounds of strength, force, and range of motion tests, they were confident that he was ready to return to practice that day—and so was he.

Granted, not everyone recovers as quickly and dramatically as Randy did. However, he's one of the thousands of patients whose experience demonstrates the power of the neurology-first approach to injury rehab, both in terms of speed and effectiveness.

As we'll discover in Chapter 3, working at the level of the brain and nervous system can also have a profound impact on patients' ability to recover from surgery.

3

THE NEUFIT METHOD FOR RECOVERING FROM SURGERY

Shortly after retiring from the NFL, former quarterback and Super Bowl champion Trent Dilfer needed total knee replacement surgery. During fourteen seasons of professional football, his body had taken its fair share of beatings.

Three weeks after surgery, Trent showed up at NeuFit headquarters. By that time, he was on a traditional post-op recovery trajectory. He felt significant pain and stiffness in and around his knee.

Though no longer playing professional football, he was still an athlete. "I was anxious to speed up my recovery," he said. "I lead an active life. Among other things, I wanted to get back to playing competitive amateur golf."

With these goals in mind, we performed our manual muscle tests and body mapping with the Neubie. In the process, we found several muscles in his leg that were practically frozen.

Due to the trauma of the surgery, we explained to him, his brain was inhibiting those muscles in an attempt to limit movement and protect his knee.

Once we pinpointed those muscles, we applied electrical stimulation with the Neubie. As we used the machine to work those areas, we asked him to do a series of simple bodyweight movements, like lunges, squats, and knee circles.

Through this combination of strategic stimulation and movement, we helped his brain and nervous system release the protective reactions, including pain and stiffness, which were standing in the way of his recovery.

"I'll never forget the first day of treatment at NeuFit," he said. "I hobbled in, barely able to walk, and the next thing I knew I had the Neubie on, and I was squatting down so far my butt was almost touching the ground!" After one session, Trent noticed big changes: his pain decreased substantially, and he gained twenty degrees of knee flexion, a fairly significant increase in range of motion.

"Between my first and second sessions, basically from one morning to the next, I went from forty very challenging revolutions on a stationary bike to pedaling an easy four and a half miles," he said. "Sure, I was hoping to recover quickly, but I never imagined I could make progress so fast."

HOW THE BRAIN RESPONDS TO SURGERY

As mentioned in previous chapters, it's not always the original trauma, but the body's response to that trauma that creates the greatest problems. This idea holds true when it comes to the body's response to surgery—even more so than after injury. (Though this is true to some extent for all surgeries, we're referring specifically to orthopedic surgeries.)

Working with thousands of clients over more than a decade, I've observed the body's responses after surgery and after injury. Based on these experiences, I'm convinced that the brain's governors, or limiting patterns, are generally more exaggerated after surgery than they are after injury.

Why does the body respond this way? Even though the body is usually in a stronger and/or more stable state after surgery, the brain doesn't understand this. It doesn't know that surgery is meant to help rather than harm.

According to the brain, the body has been attacked, torn apart, and sewn back together. As a result, the brain automatically classifies surgery as a threat—often a serious threat—to the body.

In response to this threat, the brain and nervous system send signals that inhibit, or shut down, some muscles and create excessive tension in others. Some of this inhibition comes from the brain and some from spinal reflexes.[11] Either way, it leads to atrophy in the underactive muscles and stiffness in others, slows the pace of healing, and ultimately reduces the effectiveness of the recovery process.

Trent's experience is a case in point. Immediately after his surgery, the muscles around his knee shut down and started to weaken. Three weeks after surgery, his vastus medialis oblique (the inner quad muscle just above the knee), rectus femoris (the muscle that runs straight down the thigh from the hip to the knee joint), hamstrings, and gastrocnemius (upper calf muscle) continued to deteriorate, demonstrating significant weakness in comparison to the muscles in his other leg.

During his first NeuFit treatment, however, we were able to help Trent significantly improve his strength levels in the weakened muscles of his surgical leg. To track these improvements, we used a handheld dynamometer (which we frequently use to measure the force exerted in strength tests).

The dynamometer readings in Figure 3-1 illustrate the gains Trent made during his first session. As you can see, the strength in his quad muscles increased by approximately 66 percent (from twenty-one pounds of force up to thirty-five pounds) after mapping his body and performing just fifteen minutes of neurological stimulation with the Neubie.

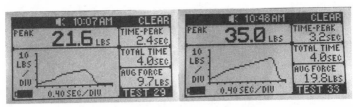

Figure 3-1: Dynamometer readings before and after Trent's first treatment.

RESETTING THE BRAIN'S RESPONSE TO SURGERY

Due to the nature of the brain's response to surgery and the amount of structural healing that needs to happen, the rehab process typically lasts longer after an operation than after an injury.

However, it's possible to reset the protective neurological patterns that tend to slow down recovery, as the example with Trent illustrates. By working at the level of the brain and nervous system, we can restore function much faster than more traditional methods of rehab and physical therapy. In the majority of cases, we can also accelerate recovery even as we reduce the risk of injury or re-injury. It all comes down to managing the neurological response to trauma.

REPROGRAMMING THE SOFTWARE TO OPTIMIZE THE HARDWARE

As with all effective forms of rehab, the neurological approach to post-surgical recovery addresses both functional and structural challenges in the body. It considers the body's hardware as well as its software, working at both levels and taking advantage of their interdependency.

In Chapter 2, we discussed the ways functional recovery facilitates structural healing after injury. The same principles apply after surgery.

In Trent's case, removing the roadblocks at the level of the brain and nervous system by stimulating the muscles around his knee freed up the body's energy to repair its physical hardware.

By shifting his body into a state to support optimal healing at the functional level, we helped it adapt more quickly and easily to the presence of the artificial knee. By upgrading his body's software, we facilitated the healing process in his body's hardware—and changed the trajectory of his recovery.

NEUFIT'S APPROACH TO POST-SURGICAL RECOVERY

NeuFit's approach to post-surgical recovery is similar to how we approach injury rehab. Though the basic principles and techniques are the same, there are two major differences in treatment after surgery:

1. It's generally more conservative.
2. It extends over a longer period of time.

Since the body is traumatized after surgery, we want to tread carefully to avoid damaging the area around the intervention. And since there's usually more structural damage, we need to allow time for the body's hardware to heal. Besides that, we sometimes need to work within movement restrictions imposed by surgeons.

So how does our approach to post-surgical rehab work in practice?

Muscle tests. Though we still want to reactivate the muscles, we generally don't perform muscle tests in exactly the same way after surgery as we do during injury treatment. If we do use muscle tests, we do them more conservatively in order to measure a patient's *pain-free* force output and strength levels.

In other words, we test to see how much they can do without any increase in pain or other symptoms. In the interest of safety, we generally do fewer tests. Ultimately, our goal with these tests is to arrive at baseline measurements that help us objectively quantify the patient's progress over the course of treatment.

If an area of the body has to be immobilized after surgery, we sometimes skip muscle tests altogether. Instead, we start treatment by applying gentle electrical stimulation to the area to increase blood flow and generate some neurological activity to minimize muscle atrophy, which can slow down the overall recovery process.

Manual muscle activation techniques. We also take a more cautious approach to manual muscle activation techniques after surgery than we do after an injury. Though these techniques vary depending on the nature of the surgery, the idea is to provide manual stimulation to help break through the brain's perception of threat in certain areas of the body to restore neurological activity and communication.

Body mapping with the Neubie. As with all rehab treatments, we typically do a full body scan with the Neubie after surgery. However, after surgery, we generally set the machine at a lower power level. This way, we make sure the electrical stimulation doesn't provoke any contractions that could cause jarring responses in the body. In other words, we want to make sure we're being as safe as possible and virtually eliminating the risk of further damage.

Applying stimulation for healing: Once we pinpoint the areas of the body where the brain is imposing guarding and limiting patterns in the form of muscle tension and/or inhibition, we gradually increase the level of electrical stimulation, just as we do in other forms of rehab.

The difference after surgery is that we generally go more slowly when ramping up the level of stimulation. And, though we still combine the stimulation with movement, these early treatments may call for less range of motion than a typical treatment since we sometimes have to work within movement restrictions. In the meantime, we constantly monitor the body's reactions to minimize the risk of a stress response that might delay recovery.

AFTER SURGERY, SAFETY COMES FIRST

Since it often leads to rapid improvements, the neurological approach to post-surgical recovery might look more aggressive or risky than traditional approaches to rehab. However, the first guiding principle for all of our work, including rehab after surgery, is to do no harm.

The neurological approach to healing takes into account the fact that the body needs time to recover after surgery. Along these lines, NeuFit always follows movement or loading restrictions prescribed by surgeons after an operation.

In some cases, we communicate directly with surgeons. In others, the patient is the go-between. No matter what form the communication takes, the goal is to make sure that everyone agrees on the course of rehab—and that patient safety comes first.

If a surgeon doesn't want a patient to bear weight on their surgically repaired leg for a certain period of time, for example, we can still make a positive impact while staying within those parameters. In this case, we have the patient perform what are called open chain movements, moving their leg while lying on a treatment table as we apply stimulation from the Neubie. This way, their recovery process still gets a boost; once they're ready to bear weight and walk again, they tend to be much further ahead than they would otherwise be.

THE ADVANTAGES OF A QUICK START TO REHAB

Why do we want to start rehab as soon as possible after an operation? As I mentioned earlier in this chapter, a patient's muscles may already demonstrate significant atrophy within a few days of inactivity.[12] This is part of why the post-surgical recovery process can take such a long time.

In fact, the more atrophy there is in the early stages after surgery, the more time and effort it takes to rebuild muscles during the late stages of the recovery process.

If we're able to start right away to stimulate the brain and nervous system to reactivate the muscles, we can reduce the time patients spend in an inhibited or shut down state after an operation. We can also reduce the amount of atrophy that tends to happen. With this approach, it often takes patients far less time to heal after an operation than if they rest for the first several weeks or even the first several days.

Both after surgery and after injury, rest may give the body time to heal, but it doesn't fix limited neurological patterns or address any of the underlying dysfunction in the body. To repair itself and grow, an adequate amount of neurological stimulation is crucial. That is, the body needs a certain level of movement and challenge to activate its recovery processes.

Recovery from injury or surgery involves all the same processes as recovery from exercise: replenishing energy, rebuilding muscles, repairing the connective tissues, and making neurological changes to adapt to the tasks performed. Because of this overlap, we can apply much of what we know about recovery from exercise in a rehab context. For one, we know that recovery is an active process that can't happen without stimulation. Research shows that the recovery systems of the body work at their peak in the period after exercise.[13] The same applies after an effective rehab session.

By contrast, when the body is at rest, it's receiving neurological signals to down-regulate and conserve energy. In this state, there's no need for the body to invest resources to adapt and regenerate by replacing what's been depleted. This describes what happens in the body when people stay immobilized after surgery.

In the process of recovering from surgery, people lose strength and function in the area of the operation. And if they don't work the other parts of the body, those areas can also get weaker very quickly. This is why it's so important to maintain all-over function after surgery.

All of this is to say that it's crucial to work toward what we call "a robust underlying physiology" in the process of recovering from surgery. After an operation, expending energy and maintaining muscle mass—not resting and being sedentary—help create the physiological conditions in the body that drive the healing process.

POST-SURGICAL REHAB: BALANCING CAUTION AND EXPERIENCE

The neurological approach to post-surgical recovery presents some exciting possibilities when it comes to increasing the speed and effectiveness of the healing process. At the same time, it's important to keep in mind that some surgical procedures require an additional layer of caution during rehab.

After procedures like supraspinatus tendon repair in the shoulder, spinal or hernia repair, and meniscus repair surgery in the knee, surgeons generally prescribe strict movement and/or weight-bearing restrictions to prevent further damage.

As mentioned earlier in this chapter, NeuFit strictly adheres to medical restrictions throughout the treatment process. At the same time, our neurology-first approach tends to shorten traditionally prescribed recovery times after surgery.

Our experience working with Katie, a softball player who tore her ACL in a skiing accident during her senior year of high school, is one of many examples that calls into question generally accepted ideas around recovery times after ACL surgery.

After the operation, Katie's doctors told her she would need at least six months to fully recover, which meant missing the entire softball season.

Since she was determined to get back on the field as quickly as possible, Katie committed to an hour of intense neurological stimulation work with the Neubie every day for three-and-a-half months. When she went back to her surgeon for an evaluation, he could clearly see that she'd regained full function.

After an exhaustive series of tests, the surgeon cleared her for play—at least two and a half months ahead of schedule. "He told me that was the earliest he's ever cleared anyone (to go back to playing sports)," Katie said.

After recovering from surgery, Katie ended up leading her high school team to the playoffs and eventually to the state championship. "I had no issues with my knee at all," she said. Then she went on to play four years of NCAA softball. "And I haven't had any issues since the surgery," she added.

Despite Katie's success story (and dozens of other stories like hers), research suggests it can take longer than originally thought for an ACL graft to completely integrate into the bone after surgery. Even if athletes reach their functional milestones more quickly than surgeons anticipate, some medical experts argue that it's important to wait before clearing them to return to play to minimize the risk of re-injury or long-term complications.[14]

If research continues to give us compelling reasons for keeping athletes from returning to the field after ACL surgery, we may revisit our approach going forward. Regardless of when they actually return to competition, we continue to see athletes reach functional milestones faster using the NeuFit Method after surgery.

SMALL VICTORIES ARE THE GOAL

Given the time it takes to reach full recovery after an operation, it's important to focus on small victories over the course of post-surgical rehab. As a former professional athlete, Trent Dilfer, whose story kicked off this chapter, understood how important these small victories were.

After his knee replacement surgery, his primary goal was to feel strong enough to play golf and restart his other physical activities without any restrictions. At the same time, he was well aware that there were lesser milestones he needed to reach on the way to those bigger goals, like incrementally increasing his range of motion and improving his strength. To reach these milestones, we created a series of easy, low-risk exercises to help him transition back into being physically active.

After a few weeks of neurological stimulation and movement therapy, Trent returned to the golf course and attempted some light chip shots. Once he could do those without any pain (and without favoring the surgical knee), we raised the level of challenge, asking him to try a fifty-yard shot. When he was able to hit dozens of those fifty-yard shots without any pain, he progressed to hundred-yard shots.

As Trent's body rose to meet each new challenge, we continued to increase the level of difficulty until he regained full function.

After two months of neurological stimulation therapy, Trent's surgeon cleared him for full play on the golf course—more than two months ahead of schedule. Though he was reluctant to clear Trent so quickly, after doing a thorough series of tests to assess flexion, extension, stability, and strength, the surgeon observed that the knee was in great shape and saw no reason to wait.

For Trent, the neurology-first approach to rehab was unlike anything he'd used over the course of his NFL career. In the end, he was so inspired by NeuFit's approach to rehab that he insisted on using it with the high school football team he coaches.

"The two biggest opponents any football coach faces are time and injuries," he said. "NeuFit solves both these problems. You take a kid that has a four-week injury, and you cut it to a one-week injury. I've seen it work on my kids, I've seen it work with me, I've seen it work with other athletes. It's truly the best technology in all of sports, development, and rehab."

As much as it can help people recover from surgery and injury, the NeuFit Method also has the potential to offer meaningful relief for people suffering from chronic pain, as we'll see in Chapter 4.

4

THE NEUFIT METHOD FOR TREATING CHRONIC PAIN

In 2017, after a relatively minor foot injury, doctors diagnosed Melinda with complex regional pain syndrome (CRPS) type II.[15]

As time went by, the pain made it practically impossible for her to function: she was homebound, confined to a wheelchair, and bedridden for all but an hour a day. "Just taking a shower would make me throw up or go into convulsions," she said. "And my foot was paralyzed."

She went from physical therapists to pain management specialists to chiropractors for help, but they couldn't do much to ease the severity of her symptoms. "The pain medications and CBD oil they prescribed gave me some temporary relief," she said, "but it was just a drop in the bucket, and it wouldn't last."

When she came to the NeuFit clinic for the first time, Melinda didn't think we could do much to help her. However, after an initial body scan with the Neubie, we could see where the pain was coming from: her brain's disproportionate reaction to the injury in her foot (as in many CRPS cases, which often start with an overreaction to a seemingly minor injury). In other words, her brain's protective response to that original injury had locked her in a cycle of extreme pain.

Starting with her first treatment, we worked to change her neurological programming. By stimulating the nerve pathways where we found blockages, we helped her brain shift its protective response.

"After one treatment," Melinda said, "I regained a bit of movement in my foot."

After her third session, she was able to point and flex her foot. Her gait started to normalize. Her flare-ups of extreme pain grew less frequent, from almost daily to one per week.

After twelve sessions, Melinda's flare-ups stopped altogether. "I'm no longer taking CBD oil or any other pain medication," she said. "I no longer have to use a cane. And the pain has completely gone away!"

THE NEUROSCIENCE OF PAIN

Melinda's experience demonstrates an important discovery about the nature of pain: pain isn't necessarily a sign that something is damaged in the body. In other words, it's possible to have damage to the body without pain, *and* it's possible to have pain without physical damage.[16]

In the past, scientists assumed that pain receptors send signals to the brain to indicate that something is wrong in the body. When a pin pricks your finger, for example, it supposedly transmits a pain signal to the brain.

However, according to modern neuroscience, here's what actually happens when a pin pricks your finger: the brain takes in that input, along with the millions of bits of input it's processing every second. Then the brain decides whether or not to create an output of pain.

Simply put, we experience pain in the brain—not in the body. In other words, pain is a neurological output signal. It's a response to what the brain perceives as a threat.[17]

Scientifically speaking, pain is a response to what neuroscientists call nociception, which is the sensory nervous system's way of signaling the presence of harmful or potentially harmful stimuli. Sometimes, these stimuli can be physical damage to the body, but sometimes they can even be psychological.

When Melinda's entire body was in pain, for example, it was her brain's way of telling her not to move, though her foot had already healed and her body wasn't actually broken.

The fact that she was able to move her foot after just one NeuFit treatment session was proof that her brain had basically shut down her body in an effort to protect it. The pain was her brain's way of saying, "That's dangerous. Don't do that."

By sending a new set of signals to her brain, we were able to reduce her brain's perception of threat. Given her body's rapid response, it was clear that her brain got the message.

EXPANDING THE WAYS TO TREAT CHRONIC PAIN

Assuming that pain means something is broken or damaged in the body limits the options for treating it. When dealing with a condition like CRPS, for example, traditional treatment methods often rely on severe medications like narcotic (opioid) painkillers, sedatives, anti-depressants, steroids, muscle relaxants, and even anesthetics.

In cases of joint or back pain, doctors and therapists frequently prescribe surgery, braces, steroidal injections, and/or non-steroidal anti-inflammatories to address the damaged hardware of the body. Again, the assumption here is that structural/hardware damage is the cause of the pain.

Obviously, if someone is in a car accident and gets injured, the body hurts at the site of the trauma. The pain has a physical cause.

However, in light of the fact that pain is a neurological response to the perception of threat, pain can actually have a diverse set of causes and circumstances—particularly chronic pain.

In cases like Melinda's, where the pain lingers long after the original injury has healed, where it comes and goes, and where it feels better at certain times of day and worse during others, it's clear that there's more to the pain than damage to the body's hardware.

If someone is suffering from chronic pain, more often than not the cause is connected to an issue in the brain and nervous system or in the body's software.

By going outside the conventional treatment toolbox, NeuFit

pinpoints the root causes of chronic pain and addresses them at the neurological level. By changing the neurological inputs, we can transform the body's outputs, especially when it comes to chronic pain.

HOW DIFFERENT AREAS OF THE BRAIN INFLUENCE THE EXPERIENCE OF PAIN

The experience of pain is connected to activity in at least twelve areas of the brain.[18] Some of these areas (e.g., the hippocampus) have to do with memory. Some are related to the emotions (the limbic region) and with projecting into the future.

Some of these brain areas are responsible for the release of stress hormones like adrenaline and cortisol (the hypothalamus). Some areas serve as a filter, deciding which inputs enter conscious awareness and which don't (the prefrontal cortex). Others have to do with things like movement planning (premotor and motor cortex), regulating sensation (thalamus and sensory cortex), and monitoring fear and threats (the amygdala).

In light of the brain's involvement in how the body processes pain, it's no surprise that there are many different elements involved in each individual's experience of pain—and that working neurologically can make an enormous difference for people suffering from chronic pain.

THE THREAT BUCKET: TRACING THE ROOTS OF CHRONIC PAIN

When treating chronic pain, we need to understand the root cause(s) in order to give patients both meaningful and long-term relief.

Again, since pain is a response to any type of threat, it's possible to trace it back to physical damage as well as to things that "shouldn't" necessarily be painful, including poor sleep quality, negative reactions to food, stress at work, conflicts with family members, or other issues and environmental challenges.

Although NeuFit treatments are primarily body-based, we find that helping patients understand both the physical and non-physical factors that contribute to pain plays an important role in overcoming it. For this purpose, we use a metaphor called the threat bucket. (The metaphor is based on the biopsychosocial model, which describes how non-physical factors contribute to pain.[19]) In the process of searching for the causes of chronic pain, we consider every possible threat and toss it into an imaginary bucket (Figure 4-1).

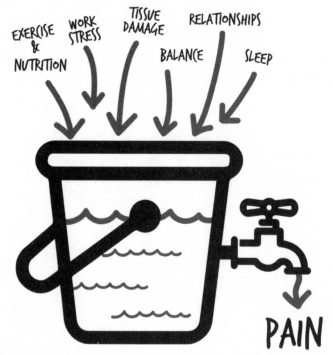

Figure 4-1: The threat bucket.

Some of these threats are physical. Others are psychological. Some are real, others imagined. At this stage, it doesn't matter what the nature of the threat is: every one of them goes into the bucket because the brain perceives every one of these inputs as a threat. And once the bucket fills up to a certain threshold, it triggers an output of pain.

For example, if a patient is dealing with an old shoulder injury that didn't heal properly or scar tissue that prevents movement in certain tissues, that goes into the threat bucket. If they have a high-stress job they're afraid to lose, or if they're having problems with their partner, we add that to the threat bucket, too. Why? From the brain's perspective, the possibility of losing a job or a partner is a legitimate threat to survival. In response to that threat, the brain may trigger a pain signal as a way to say "stop doing that" or "do something different."

When working with chronic pain patients, there are some additional questions we ask when we're trying to figure out what may be filling up their threat bucket:

- Have they had any head injuries or any physical injuries in other areas of the body that might seem unrelated to the pain?
- Do they have any scars?
- Have they had any unusual or significant stressors in their professional or personal life?
- Does the pain happen at certain times of day—or only on certain days? If so, is there something that seems to trigger the pain?
- What about their eating and drinking habits? Can they connect any changes in diet or alcohol intake with the onset of pain?

- How would they rate the quality of their sleep? Do they notice a difference in their pain level when they get a good night's rest versus when they stay up late or have trouble sleeping?

The more information we can gather from the answers to these questions, the easier it is to identify the relevant contributions to each patient's threat bucket—and work neurologically to address them.

HOW A CLINICIAN USES THE NEUBIE FOR INJURY REHAB

At the CHARM (Center for Healing and Regenerative Medicine) clinic in Austin, Texas, physical therapist and co-founder Michele Harris and her colleagues use a combination of regenerative injections and physical therapy to treat patients with chronic pain.

By helping the body repair structural damage, these regenerative treatments can alleviate some of the pain. But Harris and her fellow practitioners usually find that they need to address the other sources of threat that are contributing to the problem.

"Just because you affect and improve the structural integrity of a joint doesn't mean that someone's compensatory movement patterns or dysfunctional firing patterns miraculously get better," Harris said.

"The structural piece is really important," she continued, "but many times, neurological and neuromuscular dysfunction is what leads to degenerative joint disease or tears to begin with. With a lot of our patients, I couldn't tease away the compensatory movement patterns with the equipment I had on my hands or with other neuromuscular-based therapies."

"When I incorporated the Neubie, I saw that I could get more information about a patient's condition than I could with my other tests and assessments. The ability to scan the body and see where there's resistance or fear of loading the muscles helps us see where the dysfunction is actually located," she said.

"Being able to apply the activation signal directly to that dysfunction—as we work through the other movement patterns that we love to use—fills a major gap and takes everything in our treatment approach up by a notch or two," Harris concluded.

WHATEVER THE INPUTS, PAIN IS THE OUTPUT

Regardless of its contents, when the threat bucket overflows, the brain triggers an output signal of pain. As with protective patterns like tension and inhibition, pain is another expression of the brain and the body protecting itself. It's the brain's way of telling us to avoid moving or loading certain areas of the body.

Even if the cause is more physical than psychological, it's common for people to experience chronic pain in the same place(s) in the body. Why? If a pain signal is a response to a non-physical threat, like losing a job, there isn't a "job loss" bone or muscle where the brain can signal pain. Instead, the brain will use existing, well-rehearsed pathways to signal pain. Since the brain is constantly working to conserve energy, it doesn't make sense to invest in building an entirely new pathway for the pain. Instead, even in the case of non-physical threats, the brain sends pain signals to the same places over and over again to minimize energy expenditure.

HARDWARE- VERSUS SOFTWARE-BASED CAUSES OF PAIN

At NeuFit, besides evaluating all of the physical and psychological factors in the patient's threat bucket, we also evaluate the properties of the pain itself.

If the pain tends to vary in frequency and severity, if it's vague, and if it can't be reproduced with movement, then it's usually more software-based. That is, it's connected to or influenced by something non-physical or not specifically related to damage in the body.

The more precise the location of the pain, and the more easily we can replicate it by moving the body, the more likely it's hardware-based and related to tangible physical damage. The presence of heat, acute inflammation, and swelling are also signs of physical damage.

One of the advantages of the NeuFit Method is that it can help distinguish between the hardware- and software-based causes of pain. Software-based pain tends to resolve quickly. When pain doesn't resolve quickly, it's an indicator that there might be a hardware issue. In this case, we might need to order an x-ray, MRI, or other images. Although rare, tumors or other disease processes can also cause pain. This is part of why we want to take patients' pain seriously—and why we want to refer to other professionals when we can't completely resolve it.

TREATING PSYCHOLOGICALLY INDUCED PAIN

Is it possible to treat "non-physical" pain in a physical therapy setting? If chronic pain is rooted in something psychological rather than physical, how effective can the neurological approach be?

Even in situations where pain is related to a non-physical threat, the neurological approach to treatment still has the potential to help. Why? As we've established, whether a threat is physical or psychological, the body's response to it is still physical.

In other words, the mind isn't the only place where people process psychological threats. Remember the image from Chapter 1 of the spectators at a baseball game raising their arms to protect themselves from a foul ball? We may not react as dramatically when we perceive a psychological threat, but we do adopt elements of those same protective patterns (like a subtle contraction of the muscles in front of the body, drawing the limbs slightly inward). What's more, there's a growing body of research in the field of physiological psychology that demonstrates how psychological trauma—from post-traumatic stress disorder (PTSD) to financial, professional, or relationship conflicts—can manifest as tension and pain in the body.

For example, several studies demonstrate that factors like a hostile or uncomfortable work environment, along with job insecurity or dissatisfaction, can be significant predictors of lower back pain.[20] In cases where employees missed work due to lower back pain, researchers discovered that mechanical/physical factors weren't the main cause. Among the study's participants, higher stress levels and lower morale were more common causes of lower back pain than things like ergonomics or physical strain.[21]

Obviously, we can't change the situation at a person's job or eliminate every source of stress in someone's life. However, by working neurologically, we *can* help undo the protective physical patterns and chronic pain that result from psychological stressors.

RESTORING PROPRIOCEPTION

Another key component in addressing chronic pain at the neurological level is restoring proprioception. Proprioception is the body's overall ability to see itself in space. Put another way, it's the brain's perception or awareness of the body's position and movements.

When a patient's proprioception is compromised, it can have a dramatic effect on their brain's capacity to evaluate threats. And since pain is a response to the brain's perception of threat, it naturally follows that diminished proprioception can contribute to chronic pain.

For example, if the brain can't accurately sense where the foot is in space, as was the case with Melinda, it will interpret it as a threat. Why? Since the brain can't "see" where the foot is, it can't predict whether it might run into something or damage itself somehow.

In simple terms, having reduced or compromised proprioception is like running around with a blindfold on. When you can't see where you're going, you're much more likely to injure yourself. You also tend to move more slowly and be more guarded. In this situation, the brain often responds by locking down a limb in order to reduce movement—and minimize the threat.

Using a combination of manual techniques, joint mobility drills, and electrical stimulation from the Neubie, we increase sensory inputs in order to increase proprioception. As Melinda's experience shows, this approach can have a profound impact on chronic pain.

CHRONIC JOINT PAIN: CAN NEUFIT HELP?

Chronic joint pain is a common problem for athletes and non-athletes alike. Over the years, I've seen dozens of patients who've been told they need joint replacement surgery due to degeneration of cartilage or other joint tissues in the hip, knee, or shoulder.

How much the neurological approach can help them depends on the extent of the structural damage in the joint. In some cases, our treatment methods help patients to the point where they no longer feel pain and no longer need surgery. In other cases, the structural damage to the joint is so great that the functional approach can't make a significant difference.

In most cases, though, even the most severe structural injuries have at least some functional components. For this reason, if a patient is in line for a joint replacement, I recommend they try the neurological approach first.

For one thing, the approach is non-invasive, and the risks are extremely low. On top of that, it only takes a few sessions to assess whether or not our approach might help.

If patients don't see any tangible progress after three to five NeuFit treatments, we infer that the pain is related to a structural issue that may require surgery or regenerative treatments like injections of stem cells, plasma, or other growth factors. Though NeuFit treatments can still help as part of the recovery process, we expect it to take longer overall.

ADDITIONAL TECHNIQUES FOR TREATING CHRONIC PAIN

Even if practitioners don't have access to the Neubie, there are a series of neurologically driven strategies that can potentially help patients find relief from chronic pain.

During the assessment phase, for example, it's possible to use manual tests for sensitivity light and deep touch, vibration with a tuning fork, and sharp stimuli like a pinwheel. Two-point discrimination tests (which assess a patient's ability to detect points of contact with the skin) can also be effective to help determine the quality of sensation in an area of the body.

The point with these tests is to look for areas that are hyper-sensitive or have diminished sensitivity. The next step is to stimulate those areas—either using the test apparatus or other manual therapy techniques—to calm the hypersensitive areas and activate the deficient ones.

Besides these manual tests, monitoring skin temperature can be another valuable assessment tool in chronic pain cases. Why? Temperature changes in the limbs and outer extremities are a sign of reduced blood flow to the area, which is an indicator that the nervous system has switched into fight-or-flight mode and is activating various protective mechanisms. In this case, laser temperature sensors are the best way to ensure quick and accurate measurements of changes in skin temperature. And if there's reduced temperature in one extremity, it's time to implement a strategy to promote more activity in the parasympathetic nervous system. (We'll cover this topic in more detail in Chapters 8 and 9).

If using these muscle and temperature tests during the assessment phase, it's important to continue to use these tools throughout the treatment cycle. This way, we can accurately gauge a patient's progress and continuously monitor their neurological responses to treatment.

MANUAL MUSCLE ACTIVATION TECHNIQUES AND JOINT MOBILITY DRILLS

In addition to the manual assessments described above, it's possible to perform manual muscle activation techniques without the Neubie. These can also be helpful in restoring movement and reducing chronic pain symptoms. When used properly, these muscle activation techniques can manually break through some of the same guarding and protective patterns we address with the Neubie—and reawaken the body's dormant potential for strength and pain-free range of motion.

Since they involve pressing the thumb, forefinger, or elbow onto various trigger points, muscle activation techniques tend to take patients to the edge of their comfort zone. Part of the benefits come from the simple act of having patients breathe through their discomfort. This way, they learn to calm the nervous system—even in the face of a major challenge—and downregulate their perception of threat over time.

Strategic joint mobility drills can also help chronic pain patients, depending on the nature of the pain. Since the joints have the highest concentration of nerves of any tissue outside the brain and spinal cord, moving the joints creates significant neurological inputs. These inputs can help alleviate pain by, for example, increasing proprioception, which then reduces the level of the threat bucket.

For someone with chronic shoulder pain, for example, simple exercises like arm circles and overhead movements may expand the range of motion and reduce discomfort. In this case, mobilizing joints in other parts of the body, even as far away as the hips or the feet, can reduce the threat globally in a way that also reduces pain locally at the shoulder.

But what about someone in Melinda's condition? Could we have used manual techniques and joint mobility drills to treat her CRPS without the Neubie?

Probably. However, given the severity of her pain and the frequency of her flare-ups, it would have likely taken dozens of treatment sessions and several months to relieve her pain using manual techniques alone.

Ultimately, whether or not it involves the Neubie, the neurology-first approach can make an enormous difference in treating chronic pain. However, in the absence of strategic electrical stimulation, the results are generally not as immediate, lasting, or profound. As Chapter 5 illustrates, this holds true for patients dealing with neurological injuries or diseases as well as chronic pain.

5

THE NEUFIT METHOD FOR TREATING NEUROLOGICAL CONDITIONS

By the time she sought out treatment with NeuFit, Wendy was in a wheelchair. Thirty years earlier, she'd been diagnosed with multiple sclerosis (MS). As the disease progressed, her ability to function steadily diminished.

To slow the progression of the disease, Wendy had been using the Wahls Protocol, a version of the Paleo diet combined with other lifestyle interventions developed by the physician and medical professor Terry Wahls.[22]

"Changing my diet has definitely helped ease my symptoms," she said. "But I want to see if I can recover some of the function I've lost."

Of all the things she wanted to do again, she told us, her number one goal was being able to walk while holding her husband's hand.

With this goal in mind, we started treatment. During the first week of neurological stimulation therapy, we noticed some significant changes.

When she initially came in for treatment, Wendy couldn't move her legs at all. On her second day at NeuFit, she said, "Look what I can do!" and then proceeded to extend her left knee and lift up her foot. For the first time in at least three years, she was able to straighten her leg under her own power.

Things continued to improve from there. At the end of her third day of treatment, Wendy stopped her husband from putting on her shoes and socks for her, as he usually did. "Wait," she said, beaming, as she bent down and put them on herself. "I can't remember the last time I could do this!"

From treatment to treatment, her strength levels and ability to function continued to improve, and her confidence grew. At the end of the fifth day, she said, "I want to try and walk."

We placed her wheelchair by the front door, about eight steps away from the treatment room. Though she was limping, and though she needed her husband's arm for support, she made her way to the wheelchair on her own two feet as everyone in the office applauded.

TAPPING INTO EXISTING NEUROLOGICAL POTENTIAL

As remarkable as Wendy's experience might seem, it's not unique. Over the years, we've witnessed a number of changes like hers during treatment for a range of neurological conditions.

As we covered in previous chapters, NeuFit's treatment

approach is designed to tap into a patient's existing reservoir of physical function. For this reason, as with patients recovering from injury, surgery, and chronic pain, it can help patients coping with neurological conditions make functional changes relatively quickly.

By providing a different set of neurological inputs, our treatment methods undo patterns of learned disuse in the brain and nervous system. Learned disuse is an adaptation in which functional ability diminishes over time due to lack of activity. The following sections go into more detail on the concept of learned disuse in the context of neurological injuries or diseases.

For now, the important thing to understand is that electrical stimulation treatments like NeuFit's, which work at the level of the nervous system, have enormous potential to help improve function in many people dealing with conditions like multiple sclerosis, spinal cord injuries, traumatic brain injuries, and neuropathy, as well as patients recovering from a stroke.

Though they differ in their nature and severity, each of these conditions is rooted in an injury to the nervous system. This is why neuroplasticity is the factor that drives our treatment approach for all of these conditions.

NEUROPLASTICITY: THE KEY TO TREATING NEUROLOGICAL CHALLENGES

Thanks to the nature of neuroplasticity, or the inherent capacity of the brain and nervous system to change and adapt over time, treatments that work at the level of the brain and nervous system can be especially effective when it comes to neurological conditions.[23]

As explained in Chapter 1, our capacity for neuroplastic adaptation extends over a lifetime. Regardless of a person's age or circumstances, their brain and nervous system are capable of healing, change, and growth.[24] At the same time, it's important to keep in mind that neuroplastic changes can go in either a positive or negative direction.

How can we influence the direction of neuroplastic change? As we discussed in Chapter 1, this depends on neurological inputs. The type, strength, and frequency of neurological inputs ultimately determine whether the brain and nervous system regenerate and grow stronger or grow weaker and more dysfunctional. There are two important concepts that illustrate this phenomenon: specificity of adaptation and learned disuse.

SPECIFICITY OF ADAPTATION AND LEARNED DISUSE

Specificity of adaptation and learned disuse are key concepts that describe what drives neuroplastic change. Understanding how they work is especially important in the context of a neurological approach to rehab.

Specificity of adaptation is the notion that the brain and nervous system respond and change according to the nature of the demands on the body. In other words, specificity of adaptation is the idea that our bodies are always adjusting to get better at doing exactly what we're doing.

For example, if someone spends hours every day sitting in a hunched position over their computer, they'll actually "get better" at maintaining that posture over time. Eventually, their spine will remodel, and their nervous system will learn to hold their muscles in that stooped posture, leaving them stuck in a hunched position even when they're away from the computer.

Likewise, if someone spends hours at the gym working their biceps, they'll build strength in those muscles and along those nerve pathways (as long as they have the energy and raw materials to support those adaptations). In both cases, the specific tissues and pathways that get stimulated are the ones that adapt.

Specificity of adaptation makes it possible to rebuild damaged neural pathways as well as create new ones—so long as there's adequate stimulation (and in the sections that follow, I'll explain what "adequate" stimulation involves). In response to consistent challenges, the brain and nervous system regenerate and grow. This is the bright side of neuroplasticity.

In the meantime, learned disuse is an example of specificity of adaptation that describes the dark side of neuroplasticity. The phrase "use it or lose it" is one way to sum up learned disuse.

If someone moves certain areas of the body less and less, the brain responds by downregulating the corresponding nerve pathways.[25] As a result, these neural pathways tend to weaken over time—and the diminished nerve signals also cause muscles to atrophy. Because of learned disuse, these muscles, and the corresponding neural pathways, also lose their place in the neurological hierarchy.

In other words, since the brain's real estate is limited, and different areas of the brain are constantly competing for space, learned disuse causes underutilized parts of the brain to shut down while neighboring areas become more active.[26] The results? Patients lose strength and range of motion in the parts of the body that correspond with underused areas of the brain.

NEUROPLASTIC CHANGE TAKES TIME

Besides recognizing the bright and dark sides of neuroplasticity, it's also important to understand that neuroplastic change takes time, especially when it comes to neurological injuries or diseases.

With neurological patients, there's usually a structural (hardware) as well as a functional (software) component to the injury or challenge. And neuroplastic changes can affect both. In MS patients like Wendy, for example, sometimes the body can actually heal damaged hardware by rebuilding the myelin sheath.[27] (Myelin is the insulating layer around nerve fibers that helps them conduct signals. It's also the tissue that gets attacked by the immune system in MS patients). As discussed in previous chapters, structural changes take longer to heal, wherever they are in the body.

Wendy's remarkable progress during her first week of treatment came too quickly for any substantial structural healing to take place. The rapid nature of her improvements was a sign that they were a result of functional changes triggered by reprogramming her neurological software. In order to keep making progress, her body still needed time to repair some of the structural damage (including the damage to the myelin sheath) due to multiple sclerosis.

Over the past two years, Wendy has continued to make progress on the structural side, building strength, flexibility, and resilience. That progress is a product of hard work and consistent effort: she works out several times a week with the Neubie, week after week. She also continues to increase the level of challenge to stimulate her nervous system in new ways.

For people dealing with neurological challenges of any kind, creating positive neuroplastic changes takes a massive amount of work. As I wrote in Chapter 1, in order to achieve the amount of neural reorganization required after a stroke, for example, a patient has to invest the same amount of training time and effort as someone training to compete in professional sports. In some cases, we may not be able to repair the hardware. For any recovery to happen in these stroke or brain injury patients, the body may have to make software changes, using other parts of the brain to compensate for the damaged area(s).[28]

By integrating both the type and degree of stimulation required to drive positive neuroplastic changes, NeuFit's treatment approach can often help people achieve these changes more efficiently and effectively than conventional approaches to rehab.

REQUIREMENTS FOR POSITIVE NEUROPLASTIC CHANGE

Given that neuroplastic adaptations take time, particularly for patients with neurological challenges, what are the prerequisites for positive neuroplastic change? As we covered in Chapter 1, there are two primary requirements: a strong physiological foundation and a sufficient level of neurological stimulation.

Having a strong physiological foundation means that the body is robust and healthy enough to support neuroplastic adaptations. Factors like nutrition play a vital role here. The body needs specific proteins to build nerves and nervous system tissue. And MS patients like Wendy need high-quality fat and cholesterol in order to rebuild myelin.[29]

Besides nutrition, high-quality sleep is another crucial prerequisite for neuroplastic adaptation. What do we mean by "high-quality" sleep? It's sleep that includes sufficient amounts of deep sleep (which replenishes energy and rebuilds the bodily structures that get challenged over the course of the day) and REM sleep (which restructures the nervous system and neurological connections to integrate learning).

Chapter 9 goes into more detail about best practices for nervous system-centered nutrition, along with sleep and other lifestyle factors that impact neurological health and neuroplasticity. In the meantime, let's explore the other key prerequisite for positive neuroplastic change: adequate neurological stimulation.

DR. TERRY WAHLS ON NEUFIT'S POTENTIAL FOR TREATING NEUROLOGICAL CONDITIONS

After being diagnosed with multiple sclerosis, physician, author, and University of Iowa medical professor Dr. Terry Wahls restored her health using functional medicine and electrical stimulation therapy.

After temporarily pausing her electrical stimulation therapy treatments, she "started having a lot more trouble with back pain. So I was thrilled when I came across NeuFit, which got me back doing my e-stim [treatments], and which have become a vigorous part of my daily workout and rehab program.

"I'm so impressed with the power of electrical stimulation to change the trajectory of strengthening and rehab," she added. "NeuFit has a wonderful device, and they have partnered very well with the therapy community, [teaching them] how to incorporate electrical stimulation to accelerate rehabilitation potential."[30]

What is Adequate Neurological Stimulation?

Adequate neurological stimulation involves applying the right amount of stimulus on specific neural pathways—and applying it frequently enough to make a difference.

Why does adequate stimulation matter? In a paper titled "Observation of amounts of movement practice provided during stroke rehabilitation,"[31] researchers observed over three hundred rehab sessions with patients recovering from a stroke. Their conclusion: the amount of activity in a traditional one-hour rehab session isn't enough to drive the neural reorganization needed to restore function after stroke.

Neither the number of reps nor the difficulty of those reps was enough to drive positive neuroplastic change. Even if study participants could perform particular movements, their therapy just wasn't challenging enough to generate any meaningful improvement in those movements.

Beyond this research, what about patients who can't move certain parts of their bodies at all? If they can't do a single rep, how can they possibly perform the hundreds of thousands of reps they need to recover and improve physical function?

By stimulating areas patients can't activate on their own, the neurological approach to rehab can effectively address this challenge. With the help of electrical stimulation, we can provide the right amount and type of input to trigger the body to tap into its capacity for neuroplastic change, stimulating the body to repair damaged neural pathways and/or compensate by creating new ones. For some people, this process can actually restore movement to limbs they previously couldn't move at all.

FUNCTIONAL HEALING PROMOTES STRUCTURAL HEALING

As with all rehab patients, our goal when treating patients with neurological conditions is to optimize healing at the functional level in order to facilitate healing at the structural level.

By applying adequate neurological stimulation, we can shift the brain's resources from survival and protection to recovery and regeneration. In the process, we remove the functional obstacles that might slow down structural healing. Again, the idea is to upgrade the body's software to help the body's hardware rebuild and grow in a more efficient and effective way.

KEY AREAS OF FUNCTIONAL AND STRUCTURAL HEALING FOR PATIENTS WITH NEUROLOGICAL CHALLENGES

When treating patients with neurological injuries or diseases, NeuFit treatments may stimulate multiple types of functional and structural healing. The following is a summary of the types of functional reorganization and structural repair that our therapeutic approach can help facilitate, supporting neurological patients in restoring function and improving their quality of life.

TYPES OF FUNCTIONAL REORGANIZATION

- **Long-term potentiation** is the strengthening of existing neurological connections. Much of the function in the brain and nervous system has to do with the connections between various neurons. These connections are continuously changing in response to activity. In neuroscience, the phrase "fire together, wire together" describes this phenomenon. The idea is that neurons that fire simultaneously strengthen their connections by creating patterns that help them work together more consistently. This is part of what makes it possible to form habits, as neurological connections create "default patterns" of responses and behaviors. As with neuroplastic changes, habits can be both good and bad.

- **Brain cortex remapping** describes how certain parts of the brain take over areas that are underutilized due to learned disuse. For example, if people wear shoes with very thick soles, their brains receive fewer nerve signals from the bottoms of their feet. Over many years, the parts of the brain that monitor the feet will actually shrink because the brain isn't using them, which can lead to loss of balance and general movement deficiencies.[32] In another example, scientists who observed the brains of monkeys after severing the nerve connected to one of the monkey's fingers observed an interesting phenomenon: within just a few days, the brain areas controlling the neighboring fingers had "taken over" the brain area controlling the finger with the severed nerve.[33]

TYPES OF STRUCTURAL REPAIR

Neurogenesis describes the body's ability to create new neurons (nervous system cells) in the brain. Though it's especially crucial during embryonic development, neurogenesis continues in certain areas of the brain throughout life—and it can be a powerful mechanism for replacing damaged nerves.[34]

Axonal repair is the process of healing damage to existing neurons after traumatic injuries to peripheral nerves. Current research shows that there's little to no spontaneous axon regeneration in the central nervous system (brain and spinal cord), but scientists are working on strategies to stimulate this kind of regeneration.[35] In the peripheral nerves, however, axon regeneration does happen naturally at rates of approximately one millimeter per day.[36] In some cases, it's been shown that electrical stimulation can enhance and speed up axon regeneration.[37]

Remyelination involves the repair of the nerve tissue in the myelin sheath. With multiple sclerosis, the immune system attacks the myelin sheath, or the protective layer of tissue surrounding the nerves in the brain and spinal cord. Repairing this damage allows neurological signals to reach the extremities more easily, helping improve movement and function.[38]

WHICH NEUROLOGICAL CONDITIONS CAN BENEFIT FROM THE NEUFIT METHOD?

I've included the following stories of NeuFit patients to illustrate how our approach to treatment can help restore function and ease symptoms for people with neurological conditions such as multiple sclerosis, traumatic brain injury or stroke, spinal cord injury, and neuropathy.

MULTIPLE SCLEROSIS

Though the NeuFit Method doesn't treat the underlying autoimmune disorders that lead to MS, it can help restore function and improve quality of life by reducing spasms, providing neuromuscular re-education, increasing range of motion, improving circulation, and preventing (or even reversing) atrophy in patients with multiple sclerosis.

For patients like Wendy, combining the electrical stimulation of the Neubie with strategic movement exercises has helped improve function, increase mobility, and return to activities that were challenging or impossible before treatment.

TRAUMATIC BRAIN INJURIES

For patients who've experienced a traumatic brain injury, neurological stimulation therapy can facilitate recovery and help restore overall brain function. Diana's experience, as described by her partner Lisa, is a case in point:

> "After falling off a ladder and hitting her head on a concrete floor, Diana was in a coma for a few weeks. She spent the next seven years in rehab—and was continually frustrated because it didn't really help. Despite all that therapy, she still couldn't do things like feed herself, take a bath or get dressed.
>
> Things changed when she started working with NeuFit. Within six months, her balance improved so much that her doctors lowered her risk of falling from severe to moderate. The time it took her to walk from the parking lot to the clinic went from eight minutes to four. She can now stand without support. And her speech has improved, too."

Though it's unlikely that she'll regain full function, Diana continues to make headway: "Her quality of life has gone up more over the past six months than in the past seven years," Lisa added. Over time, her small victories have added up to meaningful progress.

STROKE RECOVERY

Besides helping people with traumatic brain injuries, NeuFit's treatment approach can also help restore function in patients who've suffered a stroke.

James, who had a stroke in his late forties and lost function in a few areas on his right side, is a prime example of someone who responded well to neurological stimulation treatments:

> "When I started treatment, I was in a wheelchair. I couldn't open my hand or straighten my arm. My speech was severely impaired, too.

> "At NeuFit, they started off by working muscles in the spots where I'd lost function. Since I was having issues with my hand, they stimulated areas in my arm and shoulder.

> "After a few months, I recovered the ability to open and close my hand on command. I could even give a thumbs up! I also got back 80 percent of my speech. After a few more months, I learned to walk again, and I even got rid of my wheelchair."

Eventually, we expect James to be fully functional on his right side again. As amazing as his progress has been, it's important to keep in mind that our ability to help patients recovering from stroke also depends on the location and severity of the brain injury. If a stroke affects multiple or large areas of the brain, or causes parts of the brain to die, then restoring functionality is more difficult—but not necessarily impossible.

SPINAL CORD INJURIES

Similar to other injury patients, people with spinal cord injuries often experience movement deficits due to two factors: 1) the trauma of the original injury and 2) learned disuse.

Working at the level of the brain and nervous system, NeuFit's approach to rehab takes both of these factors into account.

In addition to Amy's story, which kicked off this book, Matt's experience is a good example of how our treatment methods can help people with spinal cord injuries:

> "When I was twenty, I fell off an ATV and fractured my thoracic spine. After that, I was partially paralyzed from the waist down.
>
> "Before I started therapy at NeuFit, I spent three years doing regular functional electrical stimulation (FES) rehab (a popular treatment for spinal cord injuries).[39]
>
> "As long as I was hooked up to the FES machine, I could activate some of my muscles. But I still couldn't lift my leg, and as soon as they turned off the machine, I couldn't use my legs anymore."

Unlike the FES machine, the Neubie is designed to create neurological inputs that help people learn to initiate movement on their own. This is exactly what happened to Matt during his first session: "As they were scanning my body, I was able to lift my leg for the first time in ten years."

Instead of contracting the muscle for him, as with FES therapy, the Neubie tapped into his dormant neurological capacity to trigger a reflexive response. From that point on, his treatment took an upward trajectory. Besides regaining function and mobility, Matt also recovered the ability to walk again with support.

NEUROPATHY

Neuropathy—dysfunction or damage to the peripheral nerves—is similar to spinal cord injuries in that it can cause numbness, pain, tingling, and weakness. The difference is that neuropathy usually involves nerves in the extremities, especially the feet and hands.

Neuropathy can be one of the unfortunate side effects of chemotherapy and diabetes, though it sometimes shows up in people without cancer or diabetes due to infections, other diseases, or traumatic injuries. Anything that physically or chemically damages nerves can lead to neuropathy.

When treating neuropathy, NeuFit's approach focuses on helping the nerves heal and repair themselves to whatever degree the patient's body is capable. Ray's is one experience that demonstrates how effective this approach can be. Though he didn't have cancer or diabetes, he developed neuropathy when he reached his eighties:

> "Because my feet were so numb, I had trouble moving around and keeping my balance. I needed two canes to walk. And even then, it was hard for me to walk more than ten feet.

> "When I went to the NeuFit clinic, they treated me with footbaths. After about six treatments, I was walking around the block—and after a couple more treatments, I didn't need my canes anymore!"

How did this happen? Stimulating Ray's feet with electrodes under water allowed the current to disperse throughout the feet. This had a profound re-education effect, though it's difficult to know how much of the improvement was functional and how much was actually due to structural healing in the nerves themselves. In any case, the treatments cleared the path for the nerve signals to travel from his feet to his spine, which allowed his brain to more clearly perceive where his feet were.

Not all neuropathy-related treatments produce results as quickly as Ray's. However, by providing the right amount and type of neurological stimulation, we have the potential to help people recover function faster and to a greater degree than other conventional treatment methods.

NEUFIT AND NEUROLOGICAL PATIENTS: CLINICIANS' EXPERIENCE WITH NEUROPATHY

NeuFit has enabled us to show patients huge gains and immense amounts of value starting from day one.

We had one patient in particular, a very active eighty-year-old, who lifted weights, hiked, and traveled widely. That was until he had a bout of shingles, which left him with significant pain and nerve damage that forced him to use a walker.

After performing an EMG (electromyography) test, we determined that he had severe axonal damage to the L4 nerves of the spinal cord in the lower back, with the most prominent effect on the obturator nerve (which innervates the inner thigh) as a result of the shingles virus. We also noticed significantly decreased muscle recruitment. Basically, none of the motor units were firing, mostly affecting his adductors and part of the quad muscles.

We used the Neubie to strengthen the muscles with diminished nerve activity. With axonal damage in an eighty-year-old, we typically don't see significant healing or changes. But after ten months of using the Neubie two to three times per week, the patient had significant healing of the damaged axons and a completely normal EMG study.

More specifically, the EMG we did after treatment indicated collateral sprouting of the damaged axon, which shows the degree to which the Neubie was actually able to promote real nerve healing and regeneration.

Functionally, our patient is back to doing all the activities he loves. He can hike and lift weights again. He certainly doesn't need a walker. He continues to train with us two to three times per week and continues to make progress in his health and fitness.

Without the Neubie, I don't think this recovery would have been possible. And I certainly don't think he would have seen enough value to stay with us and continue to train for all those months.

—ANGELA AND JOSEPH MCGILVREY, PHYSICAL THERAPISTS AND CO-FOUNDERS
OF APEX PHYSICAL THERAPY & CONCEPTS IN REHAB IN FT. MYERS, FLORIDA

EVALUATING THE EFFECTIVENESS OF TREATMENT FOR NEUROLOGICAL CONDITIONS

The examples above demonstrate the potential of the NeuFit Method and the Neubie to help patients dealing with neurological injuries and diseases.

However, as is always the case with rehab, every patient responds differently to treatment. With some patients, the results are immediately apparent. With others, it can be more difficult to gauge whether treatment is working, how effective it is, and how effective it will be over time.

So how do we determine whether the neurological approach is the right one for treating a particular condition? The simplest way is to observe how patients respond. Most patients fall into one of three categories: fast responders, slow responders, and non-responders.

Here are some parameters for each category:

- **Fast responders** achieve tangible results within the first five sessions. These results can show up in the form of increased range of motion, higher levels of muscular control, and/or enhanced ability to perform new tasks. Meaningful increases in sensation are another sign that someone is a fast responder. Changes in the autonomic nervous system, which are observable in things like sweating in paralyzed areas of the body and blood pressure fluctuations, also indicate a fast response to neurologically focused treatment.[40]
- **Slow responders** have the same types of responses to treatment as fast responders, but it takes longer for them to reach these outcomes. In general, slow responders demonstrate at least one sign of meaningful progress between five and twenty treatments. That progress is typically enough to inspire a patient to continue treatment, especially if it's more than they've made with other therapies.
- **Non-responders** are people for whom treatment produces no reaction or improvement. If we do a body scan with the Neubie at full power and the patient doesn't feel anything, for example, it could be a sign that they're a non-responder (though this isn't always the case). In patients where the spinal cord is completely severed, or where nerves and muscle tissue have literally died, then treatment may have

little or no effect. In these cases, we hold out hope for novel therapies that may be able to help patients regenerate injured or decayed tissue.

When considering these categories, it's important to keep in mind that we usually can't know which one fits the patient until we start treatment. In too many cases—including Amy's spinal cord injury from the introduction—doctors and therapists write patients off before giving treatment a chance.

Over years of working with patients with neurological conditions, I've observed that more of them are responders than non-responders. Although we want to avoid creating false hope for patients with neurological conditions, we do want to inspire legitimate expectations. By working at the level of the brain and nervous system, we've seen many of these patients respond more quickly—and more significantly—to treatment than they imagined possible.

ALTERNATIVES TO THE NEUBIE IN TREATING NEUROLOGICAL CONDITIONS

As I wrote at the beginning of this chapter, there's an overall amount of work required to drive positive neuroplastic adaptations. For patients dealing with neurological injuries and diseases, this translates into several hours of intense, high-quality work every day. With traditional approaches to rehab and physical therapy, this intense work often goes on for years before patients experience meaningful results.

That said, there are neurological treatment alternatives to the Neubie that have the potential to help patients with neurological conditions. Techniques like constraint therapy, for example, can aid stroke recovery as well as help patients with MS.[41]

Constraint therapy involves having patients use the affected side of the body by restricting movement on the unaffected side. How does it work in practice? Take a patient who can't use their right hand. Over time, as they learn to rely more and more on their left hand, their right hand continues to lose strength and mobility due to learned disuse.

For this patient, constraint therapy would involve putting the left hand in a sling or covering it with a mitt to keep them from using it. Forcing them to use their right hand would stimulate the relevant nerves, eventually increasing function and triggering positive neuroplastic adaptations.

By driving movement in the body's compromised areas, constraint therapy can help combat the effects of learned disuse. However, constraint therapy requires a big investment of time and effort, i.e., a daily minimum of four hours, and hundreds of thousands of reps, before patients see meaningful results.

In Wendy's case, constraint therapy and/or other manual approaches to rehab may have made a difference in restoring some of the function she'd lost due to MS. But she would probably need three to five years to put in the work and see the results she achieved in her first year of neurological stimulation therapy.

Besides taking longer, manual therapies couldn't have helped Wendy regain function in areas where she'd lost it completely. In other words, manual rehab might have helped her rehabilitate some parts of her body over time, but it couldn't help her restore function where she had none.

Meanwhile, Wendy continues to make progress. "Every week," she said, "I feel like something changes for the better. Sometimes it's a little more strength in my hand. Other times it's being able to walk a few more steps. Most of the time, it's a small gain, but those little things add up." As of this writing, she's achieved her biggest recovery milestone to date: walking her son down the aisle at his wedding.

From a rehab perspective, NeuFit's treatment approach has helped make a major difference in Wendy's life and in the lives of hundreds of people with neurological conditions—as well as thousands of people dealing with injury, surgery, and chronic pain.

Now that we've covered the major types of rehabilitation, we'll turn to what happens when rehab is complete, the injury has healed, and the pain is gone. How do people transition safely and effectively from rehab to training? The answers to these questions, along with the building blocks of the neurological approach to long-term fitness and elite performance, are coming up in Part 2.

PART 2

THE NEUFIT METHOD FOR FITNESS TRAINING AND HIGH PERFORMANCE

6

THE NEUFIT METHOD FOR LONG-TERM FITNESS

Ross was at his wits' end the first time he visited the NeuFit clinic in Austin. Two months earlier, he'd undergone elbow surgery. Within the next year, he was planning to have additional surgeries on both knees, along with another on his back.

"For the last twenty years or so, I've been doing my best to try and stay in shape," he said. "The problem is my body's consistently breaking down." Chronic pain in multiple areas of his body—especially in his knees and lower back—was making it impossible for him to sustain any sort of fitness routine.

As he expressed his frustration, he told us he had two goals: "I'm a father of three, so I want to keep up with my kids. I try to get on the tennis court with them but not very successfully." As he approached his fiftieth birthday, he also wanted to train regularly, knowing how important it was to maintain muscle mass as he got older.

Over the years, Ross had experimented with a wide range of training approaches, from functional fitness and cardio to stretching and calisthenics. To relieve his pain, he'd sought out physical therapists and chiropractors.

Despite his best efforts, every time he tried to establish a workout routine, pain forced him to stop. His fitness routine was all about fits and starts: he'd work out for a couple of weeks, get injured, stop for a week, go for a week, and then be forced to take a break. It felt like a never-ending cycle.

Though he was more than ready for a new approach, he wasn't sure whether NeuFit could help him: "I came in not expecting much, and Garrett said, 'Give me three weeks and let's see what we can do.' Over the span of those few weeks, I began to feel better than I have since I was a teenager."

TRANSITIONING FROM REHAB TO FITNESS TRAINING

During the first three weeks of working with Ross, we focused on helping him recover from his recent elbow surgery and relieve his pain. Using the rehab principles covered in Part 1, we stimulated his brain and nervous system to accelerate the functional healing process.

During the body scan with the Neubie, we searched for so-called weak links, looking for the areas of his body where he demonstrated limited function due to a combination of trauma from previous injuries and bad habits. By tapping into his existing neurological potential, we helped him to let go of his brain's compensatory patterns, which were contributing to his physical dysfunction and keeping him locked in a cycle of pain.

Treating Ross's pain was one thing. Building resilience to minimize his risk of injury in the future was another. So how did we do it? And how did we decide when rehab was complete—and when he was ready to transition into fitness training?

THE DIFFERENCE BETWEEN REHAB AND TRAINING

In terms of knowing when to make the transition from rehab to training, it's helpful to keep in mind that there are more similarities than differences between the two.

Ultimately, I believe rehab is about finding areas where the brain is blocking the body's pent-up potential, using neurological stimulation to clear these blocks, and reinforcing these areas to match the functional capacity of the rest of the body.

Simply put, rehab focuses on uncovering the body's weak links and bringing them up to meet the baseline functional capacity of the body. With many patients, it's possible to reach this baseline relatively quickly. Meanwhile, training is the process of taking the baseline functional capacity of the entire system and raising it over time.

Given their fundamental similarities, there's quite a bit of overlap between effective rehab and effective fitness training. In both cases, the primary objective is to load the tissues of the body at the edge of their current capabilities, stimulating them to adapt and come back stronger. And whether someone is healing from an injury or working to raise their overall fitness level, the goals are similar from a neurological perspective: improving strength, speed, endurance, range of motion, coordination, and overall functional capacity.

TRANSITIONING FROM REHAB TO TRAINING

From a neurological perspective, the transition from rehab to fitness training is less like leaping across a chasm and more like walking up a gradual hill. At NeuFit, we don't decide rehab is "complete" when patients reach a certain milestone. Instead, we assess their progress on a continuum, steadily raising the level of difficulty as their overall functional capacity increases.

For example, once Ross reached the point where he was able to play tennis without pain, it was clear that he was ready for more challenging activities during his training sessions. With an eye toward building his long-term resilience, we continued to increase the intensity on the Neubie and raise the degree of difficulty of his exercises, along with the volume of work he was doing (i.e., the number of reps, the number of sets, and the length of various holds).

Within three months, Ross gained twelve pounds of muscle mass (according to a DEXA body composition scan) without any added hormones or supplements. Since he wasn't experiencing pain, he also decided to skip his scheduled knee and back surgeries. In the meantime, he remained injury-free. How was this possible?

Ultimately, it came down to two factors, both of which have a profound effect on any fitness training program: building resilience and enhancing the quality of neurological stimulation.

THE KEYS TO EFFECTIVE TRAINING

When it comes to training, the NeuFit Method minimizes the risk of injury and raises overall functional capacity by emphasizing two primary elements of training:

1. **Building nervous system resilience,** or developing physical and psychological capacity to handle increasing levels of challenge without being thrown off course.
2. **Enhancing the quality of neurological stimulation** to optimize the processes of remodeling, repair, and growth at the physiological level.

How exactly do we address these aspects of training? It starts with understanding the general hierarchy of the nervous system. Knowing how the nervous system works gives us the tools to build resilience, provide the optimal level of nervous system stimulation, and help people raise their fitness levels and boost their health over the long term.

THE HIERARCHY OF THE NERVOUS SYSTEM

The nervous system is divided into three states: parasympathetic, sympathetic, and frozen.

In a parasympathetic state, also known as "rest-and-digest" or "feed-and-breed," the nervous system distributes energy and other resources to activities that promote the body's long-term repair and growth processes. In this state, blood pressure is under control, and the organs associated with digestion, elimination, and reproduction have plenty of energy to function optimally.

When there's an increase in stress or challenge, the parasympathetic nervous system gets overwhelmed, and the sympathetic nervous system takes over. This is also known as the "fight-or-flight" response, which is a major part of the brain's survival mechanism.

Whenever the brain perceives danger, the sympathetic nervous system automatically kicks in. This is how our bodies mobilize energy to meet immediate challenges, releasing hormones like adrenaline and cortisol, increasing heart rate and blood pressure, and moving energy from the visceral organs out to the major muscles, fueling them to fight an attacker or flee from danger.

When the sympathetic nervous system gets overwhelmed, the nervous system reverts *back* into a parasympathetic state. In these situations, we go to the opposite side of the parasympathetic system, into what's known as the freeze response. What does this look like? Fainting is the most extreme freeze response, e.g., when someone passes out before they go on stage or when they see a needle during a medical procedure.

The freeze response kicks in when the brain perceives a serious and immediate threat to survival, seeing no other choice but to shut down, feign death, and hope to wake up on the other side.

THE TWO BRANCHES OF THE PARASYMPATHETIC NERVOUS SYSTEM

Does it seem like a paradox that the parasympathetic nervous system's "freeze" response has such a different effect than the "rest-and-digest" response? Stephen Porges, Ph.D., explains the physiology behind this apparent paradox in his book *The Polyvagal Theory*.[42]

According to Dr. Porges, the vagus nerve, the main pathway by which the parasympathetic nervous system regulates the visceral organs, actually has two branches—and these two branches function very differently.

The first one, the ventral branch, is the "higher level," more recently evolved branch that regulates the body when things are generally under control. Activity in this branch of the vagus nerve leads to high heart rate variability, which is a significant measure of health and resilience.

When the parasympathetic nervous system gets overwhelmed, the sympathetic nervous system takes over as the next stage in this hierarchy.

Then, when the sympathetic nervous system is overwhelmed, it's the other branch of the vagus nerve—the dorsal branch—that takes over. This is also known as the "reptilian branch" in the more primitive parts of the brain, and it triggers the freeze response. (A common manifestation of the freeze response is fainting, which is often referred to as the vasovagal response.)

WHAT DOES OPTIMAL NERVOUS SYSTEM FUNCTION LOOK LIKE?

Given the hierarchy of the nervous system, what does optimal nervous system function look like?

When it comes to nervous system health, the goal is to shift between states of (sympathetic) high activity and (parasympathetic) rest and recovery *as often as necessary* to reach our health and fitness targets.

When there's a problem at the level of the nervous system, it's not because any of the states are inherently unhealthy. Problems come up when we get locked in any one state for too long.

Spending too much time in a sympathetic-dominant state, for example, leads to the production of stress hormones that can cause long-term health problems. However, excessive parasympathetic nervous system activity can be harmful, too. Why? If we never step outside our comfort zones or challenge our bodies, then we take away the opportunity to grow and improve. As a result, our bodies end up weakening over time.

Here's the bottom line: during periods of high output and immediate challenge, we want the body to move into a sympathetic-dominant state. During periods of recovery and regeneration, the aim is to be in a parasympathetic-dominant state, where the body channels resources toward replenishment and long-term growth.

CORTISOL AND THE NERVOUS SYSTEM

Another way to understand optimal nervous system function is to look at it in the context of cortisol levels. As a stress hormone, cortisol is valuable in mobilizing energy to meet immediate challenges. However, it can have negative consequences when it stays in the system for too long.

The following graph, adapted from *Why Zebras Don't Get Ulcers* by Robert Sapolsky,[43] uses cortisol levels to show how the nervous system responds to stress:

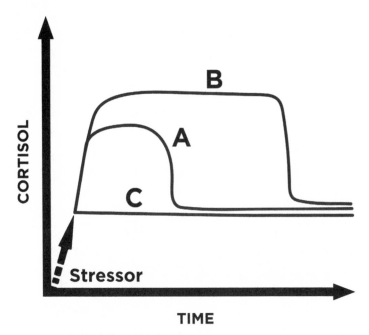

Figure 6-1: Cortisol levels demonstrate how the nervous system reacts to stress.

In this graph, line A is the goal. Following line A, the sympathetic nervous system rises to meet a challenge, like a workout or a high-stakes situation. Once the person has dealt with that challenge, the parasympathetic nervous system takes over, allowing the body to replenish energy, restore balance, and rebuild muscle as it recovers. This is a healthy cortisol response. This is how we want the nervous system to function.

Line B represents an unhealthy cortisol response, not to mention one of the most common health problems in modern society: remaining in a stressed-out, fight-or-flight state for too long. This is what it looks like when the sympathetic nervous system gets triggered and can't find its way back to rest-and-digest mode. In this state, cortisol levels go high and stay high.

Line C in the graph represents someone who remains in a parasympathetic state (i.e., at a low cortisol level), regardless of the stress or challenge. This low cortisol level can indicate a freeze response, where the nervous system is so depleted it's unable to mount a response to a stressor. At the other extreme, it can also indicate a high level of nervous system resilience, as in a Special Forces operator in the military who's trained to respond to challenges without relying on a jolt of stress hormones.

If line A in the graph is the goal, what can we do to condition the body for a healthy cortisol response—and help the nervous system function at an optimal level?

It starts with building resilience, or increasing the threshold for transition between the parasympathetic and sympathetic nervous systems. The greater this threshold, the easier it is for the body to handle stress and challenges and remain in a healthy neurophysiological state. This allows the body to save its sympathetic resources for when they're truly needed.

BUILDING RESILIENCE FOR OPTIMAL NERVOUS SYSTEM FUNCTION

When it comes to training, building resilience is at the core of the NeuFit Method. However, before we explore best practices around building nervous system resilience, it's important to clarify what we mean by resilience in the context of a neurological approach to fitness training.

As I wrote earlier in this chapter, resilience is defined as the ability to handle more significant levels of load or challenge without being thrown off course. In terms of training, being thrown off course could mean getting injured (or re-injured).

It could also mean compensating in movement or body position, as when someone is lifting too much weight in a bicep curl and has to arch their back to pull the weight to the top of a rep.

Psychologically, being thrown off course involves losing focus, having a short temper (and reacting to certain situations in ways we later regret), or "choking" in a high-pressure situation, on or off the field.

To help people stay the course, our training approach focuses on increasing the level of load and challenge while minimizing the risk of injury. Working from the client's baseline capacity, we methodically raise the functional capability of their entire system over time—all in the interest of building resilience.

DIMENSIONS OF RESILIENCE

When it comes to training, the concept of resilience is fairly straightforward. At the same time, our training methods integrate several different dimensions of resilience. These include strength, resistance to injury, resistance to environmental stressors (like temperature changes), and the capacity to deal with psychological stress (i.e., mental resilience).

Building Resilience with Strength

As a key dimension of resilience, strength is the neurological ability to contract large amounts of muscle at the same time. To put it another way, it's the sum of individual muscle fibers working together to create force.

The average person can only contract 30 percent of their existing muscle at any moment in time.[44] Why? Again, this goes back to the brain's survival mechanism. The brain and nervous system want to keep the muscles from contracting too hard in order to minimize the risk of injury. This neurological reflex is an important safety mechanism, but it often sets the body's threshold too conservatively, limiting its ability to tap into dormant reserves of strength.

With Ross, as we do with most of our training clients, we focused on building strength in two ways. First, we worked on re-education to increase muscle recruitment, gradually changing the settings on the Neubie to create more activation in the muscles than he could create on his own. By increasing the load over time, we helped him draw on more of his existing muscle fibers. In the process, we also taught his brain and nervous system that it was safe to use more of his available strength. (This is also known as enhancing intramuscular coordination.)

Besides boosting Ross's capacity for muscle recruitment, we also accelerated the process of hypertrophy, or the building of new muscle. Why does hypertrophy matter? Not only does it contribute to functional capability, but it also becomes increasingly important as people get older. Since muscle is a metabolic and hormonal engine, maintaining muscle mass is a crucial part of aging gracefully (see the callout box).

With traditional approaches to training, building strength and hypertrophy usually require that people lift heavier and heavier weights. Though weights can be beneficial, they also increase the risk of injury.

In contrast, when we work at the neurological level, we can

increase the challenge by combining electrical stimulation with simple but strategic movements—and less external load. In Ross's case, doing targeted exercises like body weight squats and isometric lunges while being hooked up to the Neubie helped him reach his strength goals without touching a weight.

STRENGTH, MUSCLE MASS, AND HEALTHY AGING

There are several studies that establish a meaningful connection between greater muscle mass, longer life, and better overall health in older adults.[45] There's also evidence that electrical stimulation can induce positive changes in the muscles of elderly people, making them stronger and more supple.[46]

Whichever training method people choose, the good news is that there's no age limit in terms of their capacity to build muscle through strength exercises and workouts. [47]

As the body's biggest burners of energy, muscles are crucial for metabolism. This is why someone with more muscle mass will have a higher metabolism than someone with less. What's more, muscles help control blood sugar. With the support of insulin, the muscles pull in glucose from the blood and lower blood sugar levels.

Muscles are also important from a hormonal perspective. Having more muscle means having more anabolic hormones like testosterone and growth hormone, which facilitate protein synthesis and new tissue formation.

Conversely, greater levels of fat and lower levels of muscle are associated with higher levels of stress hormones and inflammation, which can lead to a variety of health issues and diseases, including arthritis, cancer, diabetes, and autoimmune disorders.

When it comes to muscles and hormones, it's ultimately a two-way street: better hormones lead to more muscle mass, and having more muscle mass supports the production of better hormones.

Building Resilience through Resistance to Injury

Besides building general strength, training the body to resist injury—especially in specific situations and in specific positions—is another important dimension of resilience that we incorporate into our training at NeuFit.

What does this look like in practice? If Ross is on the tennis court and he changes direction, for example, this puts quite a bit of lateral tension on the ankle ligaments. In this situation, if he rolls his ankle and it can't handle that tension or force, then he runs the risk of injuring himself.

Fortunately, we can work toward preventing these types of injuries by challenging the muscles and connective tissues and training them to handle higher levels of force. When he started training with NeuFit, for example, Ross's ankle might have been able to manage 150 pounds of force before its ligaments would tear.

Over time, using strategic mobility drills that load the ligaments and connective tissue in the inversion position, his ankle reached the point where it could handle significantly more force, say 250 pounds. (This is due to a phenomenon called Davis's Law—another aspect of specificity of adaptation—that describes how connective tissues adapt and remodel to meet the body's demands.[48])

Now that he can handle higher levels of force in his ankle, Ross is much less likely to roll or invert it the next time he changes direction on the tennis court—and much less likely to be injured if he does roll it. In other words, his capacity to handle more force translates into greater resistance to injury.

Building Resilience to Environmental Stressors

Building resilience through activities like cold exposure is another useful tool for training the nervous system and the body to better handle stress. Besides reducing inflammation[49] and helping improve the metabolism,[50] cold exposure—in the form of ice baths, cold showers, cold water swimming, and/or cryotherapy chambers—is a powerful technique for increasing the threshold between the sympathetic and parasympathetic nervous systems.[51]

Exposure to cold temperatures usually causes the nervous system to start panicking and shift into fight-or-flight mode. If someone jumps into an ice bath, for example, their brain's first reaction is to perceive the freezing temperature as a threat to survival. In response, the body releases stress hormones and redistributes blood, moving it away from the extremities and into the organs to preserve its core temperature. Though this is a healthy physiological response, the goal is to be able to redistribute blood using only the necessary amount of sympathetic response—and no more than that. In simple terms, the goal is to react, not to overreact.

With cold exposure therapy, we can learn to manage this

threat response by teaching the nervous system to respond differently to changes in temperature. Instead of panicking in the ice bath, intentionally slowing down the breathing and consciously calming the mind builds the nervous system's capacity to handle greater levels of challenge and stay in a healthy parasympathetic state. With training, people can learn to handle cold exposure without having a major fight-or-flight response and calling upon reserves of stress hormones. As mentioned earlier in this chapter, this allows them to reserve these hormones for situations when they need them most.

There are various ways to incorporate cold exposure into training. Twenty to thirty seconds in the shower are generally enough to get started. For Ross, the occasional cold shower was effective. Eventually, he worked up to spending one or two minutes in his backyard swimming pool in the winter.[52]

ADDITIONAL EXERCISE TECHNIQUES FOR STRENGTH AND RESILIENCE: YIELDING ISOMETRICS AND END RANGE ACTIVATIONS (ERAS)

Yielding isometrics and ERAs are manual exercise techniques that build resilience by increasing strength, endurance, and range of motion while simultaneously decreasing injury risk.

Though they're more effective when combined with the electrical stimulation of the Neubie, both yielding isometrics and ERAs can be beneficial when practiced on their own.

ERAs and yielding isometrics are similar in that they both build resilience by intentionally training through a fatigued state (and doing it in a safe and controlled way). The main difference between the two is that

ERAs involve starting in the lowest position while yielding isometric exercises start in the highest position.

How exactly do these exercises work? Through long holds of strategic positions, both ERAs and yielding isometrics trigger greater muscle recruitment than traditional body-weight exercises.

In the beginning, a portion of the available motor units activate, signaling the associated muscle fibers to contract. As time goes on, the first groups of muscle fibers churn through their existing energy supply, and fatigue sets in. The body responds by calling on additional motor units in the muscles to handle the load. Eventually, as fatigue builds, the body calls on the most powerful motor units, which typically only activate when lifting heavy weights.

Figure 6-2 shows how the muscle recruitment process plays out over the course of an exercise:[53]

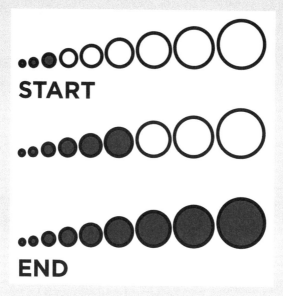

Figure 6-2: Increasing motor unit recruitment during exercise.

In the later stages of these exercises, it's common to feel (and see) the muscles shaking. This shaking is to be expected since it's part of the subtle shifts between the areas of the muscles bearing the load. Assuming it's not due to any underlying health issues, shaking is a sign of increased neurological output and activation of a broad range of motor units and muscle fibers within that muscle group.

Both ERAs and yielding isometrics provide many of the same benefits as heavy lifting. At the same time, they minimize the risk of injury in two ways:

- By training eccentric muscle contractions, in which the muscle fibers learn to lengthen to protect the body, as they do during the deceleration phase of movement.[54]

- By creating muscle activation throughout the entire range of motion, especially at the end ranges where the body has the least amount of control. This trains the muscles to protect the body in the ranges where it's most vulnerable to injury.

Chapter 7 goes into more detail about the importance of eccentric muscle contractions for preventing injury. In the meantime, here are a few examples of yielding isometric and ERA exercises (visit www.neu. fit/book for more instruction on ERA and yielding isometric exercises, along with a sample workout):

- **The Two-Minute ERA Lunge**: This exercise is partially inspired by martial arts traditions, in which practitioners hold certain positions (e.g., horse stance) for long periods of time to promote vitality and resilience. As an ERA exercise, holding the bottom of a lunge position for two minutes (or more) is a safe way to increase the level of challenge while increasing endurance and strength, particularly in the lower body. The goal is to actively attempt to sink lower and lower in the lunge throughout the exercise, so the muscles continue to lengthen and actively stabilize the joints for the entire duration.

- **The Two-Minute Push-up**: This exercise involves holding the bottom of a push-up position, working up to two minutes initially, and progressing to longer holds over time. Like the lunge, it's a hold at the bottom position with an intention to continue lowering the body throughout the exercise. Since doing it on the floor limits the range, it's best to practice it with the hands on a chair or a handle of some sort, which makes it easier to lower the body even further.

- **The Two-Minute Yielding Isometric Shoulder Raise**: This shoulder-training exercise involves holding light dumbbells—often just two to three pounds—while extending the arms to the front or the side. When the arms start to fatigue, they naturally drop. Instead of raising them again, the idea is to continue to hold the arms in the lowered position. This helps promote eccentric muscle contractions, which strengthen the muscle fibers in a way that increases their ability to resist injury.

Building Psychological Resilience

In addition to the physical aspects, psychological resilience is another important dimension of resilience. The ability to stay cool under pressure is one of the keys to optimal nervous system health, whether you're a basketball player at the free-throw line with a championship game at stake or a business executive on the cusp of a game-changing deal.

Special Forces operators like Green Berets and Navy SEALs—who endure months of grueling training to condition their nervous systems for life-threatening situations—are examples of a population with extremely high levels of psychological resilience. At the other end of the spectrum, many monks who spend their lives in meditation can also reach extraordinary degrees of mental resilience.

Though their methods and goals are different, both special operations soldiers and monks train themselves to handle scenarios that would trigger a stress response in the average person. That is, they develop the capacity to meet high-stakes challenges and psychological events without shifting into fight-or-flight mode.

Granted, most people don't experience the types of situations a monk or a special operations soldier deals with on a regular basis. At the same time, the ability to handle stress neurologically is a key component of overall fitness for everyone. Why?

When we build psychological resilience, we also build our capacity to take on greater levels of challenge while remaining healthy and fit over the long term. At NeuFit, two of the primary ways we help clients build this capacity are through using the Neubie and controlling the breath.

Using the Neubie to Build Psychological Resilience

When using the Neubie during a rehab or training session, there are times when we raise the power levels to the point where they push clients outside their comfort zone. In the face of discomfort, the lower parts of their brains start to panic, and most people naturally want to stop or quit.

However, if we can coach people to breathe and move through the current, an amazing thing starts to happen: they adapt to the current instead of fighting against it. Each time this happens, clients learn that they're capable of handling more challenges than they previously thought. Over time, this process leads to positive neurological adaptations, including greater psychological resilience. The breath is key to facilitating these adaptations.

Breathing for Psychological Resilience

The way a person breathes plays a major role in nervous system function and in the body's stress response. Through the simple practice of nose breathing—especially during exercise, when it's most challenging—we can train the nervous system to handle increasing levels of stress while remaining in a healthier, parasympathetic-dominant state.

Why does nose breathing make such a difference in nervous system function? It goes back to the idea of specificity of adaptation. In other words, the body responds and adapts to exactly what a person is doing.

Imagine, for example, that someone takes a twenty-minute run. The run can be helpful or harmful depending on how they do it.[55] If they're practicing good posture, breathing in and out through the nose, and focusing on slowing down the breath while they're running, they're essentially teaching the body to stay calm in the face of stress. This way, even though their heart rate is increasing and they're challenging the body's energy systems, their nervous system doesn't shift as significantly into fight-or-flight mode to meet the challenge.

On the other hand, if they go on a twenty-minute run and spend the entire time hunched over, panting, and breathing through the mouth, they're actually training the nervous system to be in fight-or-flight mode. (By itself, mouth breathing signals the nervous system to shift towards fight-or-flight.) As a result, their body adapts to being in this state, signaling the nervous system to lock into sympathetic mode for the rest of the day.

Chapter 9 goes into more detail about how to use breathing to improve nervous system function, including various breathing techniques and a deeper discussion on breathing mechanics, oxygen, and carbon dioxide. For now, it's important to keep in mind that practicing nose breathing during training—by intentionally overriding the impulse to breathe through the mouth—is one of the best ways to build resilience, both physical and psychological.

ENHANCING THE QUALITY OF NEUROLOGICAL STIMULATION IN TRAINING

Besides taking a multi-dimensional approach to building resilience, the other crucial component in NeuFit's approach to training for general health and fitness is enhancing the quality of neurological stimulation.

Many conventional training programs limit their focus to the muscles or the cardiovascular system, paying little attention to the neurological effects of what they're doing. However, when we enhance the quality of neurological stimulation, we can have a more profound effect on long-term fitness. How? By facilitating continuous regeneration and growth at the physiological level.

In order to kickstart these beneficial physiological processes, training has to be stimulating or strenuous enough to trigger the body's recovery mechanisms. Why does recovery matter?

Recovery is when the so-called magic happens at the level of the nervous system. In other words, training itself doesn't improve health and performance. Instead, *it's the adaptations that happen during recovery from training that provide the health and performance benefits.* During recovery, the body replenishes depleted energy stores. It also starts to rebuild and reinforce damaged structures—for example, strengthening and/or building muscle—in order to adapt and be able to perform better next time.

When recovery is at its peak, the metabolic rate increases to fuel the recovery process, and the body optimizes its hormonal profiles. Essentially, peak recovery is when we experience the true benefits of exercise. Unfortunately, most people who work out never actually take full advantage of these benefits.

Standard weekly exercise routines, which might include three cardio workouts plus a few weight machines at the gym, rarely create enough neurological stimulation to activate the body's recovery mechanisms, let alone drive them to function at full capacity. Too often, people get stuck in the same workout routine. Despite exercising for years on end, their bodies don't change—at least not for the better.

Although some exercise is certainly better than none, the average workout is usually not enough to send a signal to the brain that something meaningful has happened in the body (i.e., that the body has overcome a challenge). Without this signal, the nervous system can't shift as completely (or as significantly) into parasympathetic mode after a workout, where it engages in the repair and remodeling processes that promote long-term health and fitness.

WHAT DOES OPTIMAL RECOVERY LOOK LIKE?

When we train optimally, we also recover optimally. These are the five important physiological processes that take place during an optimal recovery cycle,[56] in the approximate order they take place:

1. **Restoring energy**, including adenosine triphosphate (ATP), creatine phosphate, and glycogen.
2. **Normalizing water and ionic balances**, or water and electrolytes within the cells.
3. **Removing metabolic waste** so the body can better absorb the nutrients it needs. This process also helps clear unwanted buildup, like plaques in the body or brain that can lead to long-term problems.
4. **Rebuilding cellular structures** that were challenged during exercise, like muscle fibers, tendons, ligaments, and bones, so they grow stronger and can withstand future challenges more effectively.
5. **Remodeling the nervous system** to strengthen specific synaptic connections and/or create new nerve pathways. (These adaptations are specific to the neurological pathways challenged during a training session.)

WHEN IS A WORKOUT STIMULATING ENOUGH?

In reality, it's difficult to know in advance whether a workout will be stimulating enough to promote optimal nervous system function and kickstart the body's recovery processes.

When we're designing training programs at NeuFit, we start off by evaluating a client's current capacity, using the information gathered from muscle tests, body scans with the Neubie, and observations of performance in various activities. Once we have this information, the goal is to challenge that client's current capacity in order to raise their baseline fitness level by applying the right type and amount of neurological stimulation.

After each workout, we use a series of indicators to gauge the client's neurological responses to training (Chapter 8 goes into detail about the key indicators of nervous system function and health).

Based on factors like heart rate variability, blood pressure, energy level, bowel function, and psychological status, we can judge whether a workout was stimulating enough to shift the nervous system into a parasympathetic-dominant state.

If a workout isn't stimulating enough, or if it provides too much stimulation, then the nervous system tends to stay in sympathetic mode, keeping the client locked in a stressed-out state long after they finish exercising.

One way to ensure that workouts are sufficiently stimulating is to use a tool like the Neubie, which significantly yet safely raises the level of challenge. This way, clients benefit from increasing neurological and physical stimulation and reduce their risk of injury at the same time.

In contrast, traditional training approaches usually require that people do things like lift heavier weights, run faster, or exercise longer to increase the intensity and effectiveness of a workout. Although these activities have a place in training for athletic performance, they also increase the likelihood of injury and may not be appropriate for general fitness training clients (or anyone who's not adequately prepared).

In cases where we want to incorporate some of these more traditional training methods, there are options and tweaks that can make them more effective neurologically. For example, some of the latest science on cardiovascular training explores strategies like interval training, which can improve traditional cardio workouts by making them more neurologically stimulating as well as more efficient.

THE BENEFITS OF INTERVAL TRAINING

Does exercising longer improve nervous system and heart health? Not necessarily. And these improvements also depend in large part on *how* people exercise.

For most people, short bouts of exercise at maximum or near-maximum capacity—also known as interval training—provide the same (or even greater) general health and cardiovascular benefits as long periods of cardiovascular exercise.

According to researchers at McMaster University in Ontario,[57] two minutes of maximum effort during exercise affects mitochondrial biogenesis (a key source of aerobic energy and a major influence on long-term health) as much as thirty to sixty minutes of aerobic training.

Other studies go even further,[58] stating that a couple of maximum-effort bouts lasting just twenty seconds can have the same health benefits as a thirty-minute workout.

With interval workouts, people can achieve more benefits, or at least the same amount of benefits, in much less time than a typical cardio workout. For example, doing a series of short sprints and allowing the body to recover completely between bouts generally stimulates both the nervous and cardiovascular systems more than jogging three miles at a light, steady pace.

ENHANCING NEUROLOGICAL STIMULATION THROUGH MOBILITY EXERCISES

Taking the joints through their full range of motion is another critical component of effective fitness training. Why? If people only focus on building muscle during training, they run the risk of becoming stiff and inflexible over time.

Outside of training, when it comes to movement, most people have a habitual range in which they use their bodies. Take the arms, for example. Most of the arms' activities—like typing, driving, eating, and cooking—are right in front of the body. It's rare for many people to use their arms for much else. Generally speaking, they don't move their arms overhead, to the side, or behind them.

Due to the specificity of adaptation and the "use it or lose it" principle, range of motion grows increasingly narrow over time—unless we take action (i.e., do exercises) to preserve or expand it.

Besides increasing flexibility, mobility exercises also help enhance the quality of neurological stimulation during workouts. How? Remember that the joints have an extremely high concentration of nerves. Moving the joints through their full range activates nerve receptors and increases signals from the joints, creating neurological inputs that significantly activate the nervous system and help trigger optimal recovery. Taking all the joints (including the hips, knees, ankles, feet, spine, shoulders, elbows, and wrists) through their full range of motion on a regular basis also reduces the risk of injury and loss of function over time.

In the context of fitness training, joint mobility drills, or movements that push the body beyond its usual movement patterns, are one of the best ways to expand range of motion—and give the brain and nervous system the type of stimulation they need to function at their peak. (At www.neufit.com/book, I share mobility drills to use as warm-ups before training or as part of a routine to improve long-term joint health.)

EFFICIENT TRAINING FOR SUSTAINABLE RESULTS

With any fitness approach, it takes time for the body to make meaningful adaptations and improvements. However, training at the neurological level can significantly accelerate this process. When a workout is neurologically stimulating and triggers effective recovery afterward, clients can overcome their plateaus more effectively and often make progress in each session. This helps them achieve results in far less time than with conventional approaches to training.

This was certainly true for Ross. After three NeuFit sessions, he was able to walk down the stairs without any knee pain at all (even though he was scheduled for knee surgery). Within three weeks, he went from holding a lunge for thirty seconds to holding it for three minutes. For the first time in more than a decade, he was able to play tennis injury-free.

Five years after his first treatment, Ross still trains with us every week. "I have no pain," he said. "And at age forty-seven, I feel better than I did in my twenties."

Ross's experience is just one example of the power and potential in the neurological approach to training. Besides giving him a safe, effective, and efficient workout structure, it helped him build a foundation for lifelong fitness and health.

Beyond general health and fitness, working at the level of the brain and nervous system also has great potential when it comes to improving athletic performance. As Chapter 7 illustrates, integrating a neurological focus into their training can give high-level athletes a considerable edge—and help them maintain that edge over the long term.

7

THE NEUFIT METHOD FOR ELITE ATHLETIC PERFORMANCE

After seventeen years in the NHL, all-star defenseman Brent Burns felt himself slowing down. The grueling eighty-two-game season—along with frequent travel, lack of sleep, and the injuries that come with playing professional hockey—were taking an increasing toll on his body.

As an elite athlete, Brent was constantly looking for ways to improve his performance: "I'm always interested in trying to better myself and prolong my career as long as possible," he said. "When I saw the (Neubie) machine, I knew right away that it could help me."

At age thirty-three, he decided to incorporate the Neubie into his training regime as part of his preparation for the 2018 NHL season. "As I've gotten older, it just takes longer to get ready to work out," he said. "So when you find something that can get you there faster and feeling stronger than you can by yourself? It's a win."

"(My warm up) usually takes me forty-five minutes to an hour," he added. "With the machine, I'm ready to go in five to ten minutes." Instead of manually rolling out the muscles and slowly ramping up the intensity as in a traditional warm-up, the stimulation from the Neubie helped his body go through the same process in a much shorter period of time. How? By increasing blood flow and quickly activating the muscles he used on the ice.

Besides helping him warm up faster, neurological stimulation improved the precision and efficacy of his workouts: "My hips feel looser. And in the workouts, I'm crushed a lot faster!" he said with a smile. "And there's no way to cheat around the system. It gets that whole hard drive pumping. Incorporating all the muscles to work properly. It's incredible."

THE NEUROLOGICAL APPROACH TO ELITE PERFORMANCE TRAINING

Like rehab and general fitness training, athletic performance is highly dependent on the brain and nervous system. Since the brain's first priority is survival, its protective mechanisms often set the body's limits too conservatively, "hitting the brakes" in moments of exertion and unnecessarily reducing performance to prevent injury.

Brent's experience is a powerful example of how we can use targeted neurological interventions to change the brain's software programming. When we change this programming, we can release limiting patterns driven by the brain's survival bias and significantly improve athletic performance.

By combining electrical stimulation from the Neubie with strategic mobility drills and other general and sport-specific exercises and techniques, we can help athletes perform at their peak. In addition, we can enhance their ability to sustain peak performance and maximize their individual genetic potential. (As the callout box explains in more detail, performance isn't completely dependent on genetics.)

WHAT ROLE DOES GENETICS PLAY IN ATHLETIC PERFORMANCE?

When it comes to athletic ability, it's common for people to assume that they're prisoners of their genes. However, according to sports scientist Michael Yessis, Ph. D., **only 30 percent of athletic potential is genetic**. The remaining 70 percent is based on environmental factors like training, nutrition, and lifestyle decisions.[59]

The truth is the majority of athletes never actually reach their full genetic potential. Why? It comes down to two factors:

- **Training**: Training too little or too much, not training consistently for a sufficient amount of time to achieve long-term progress, and/or not training in a way that stimulates positive neurological and physical adaptations.

- **Lifestyle**: Poor eating and/or sleeping habits, along with other lifestyle choices (like drinking excessive amounts of alcohol) that diminish the body's ability to recover outside of training.

Take an athlete with a high genetic ceiling who doesn't train long or hard enough to reach it. When they compete against an athlete with a little less natural talent who trains harder and smarter, they lose most of the time.

Ultimately, the ideal combination is the best genetics coupled with the best training and lifestyle. But I find Dr. Yessis's message—that it's still possible to achieve high levels of performance even without the best genes—both inspiring and accurate.

PREPARING THE BODY FOR OPTIMAL PERFORMANCE

Many athletes assume they need to spend the majority of their training time practicing the skills unique to their sport. But here's the bottom line: it's difficult to get the full benefits from directed skill work without first laying a foundation of basic movement proficiency, endurance, strength, and speed.

In other words, before a hockey player like Brent Burns can master skills like skating, passing, and shooting, he needs to train his body to move efficiently, handle stress well, and effectively recover from a challenge. Since all of these attributes are neurological in nature, we can develop and strengthen them by working at the level of the nervous system.

Without this neurological work, the benefits of doing focused skill training are limited. Sooner or later, athletes hit an artificial ceiling when it comes to their progress. This artificial ceiling can manifest in a variety of ways: a tendency toward injury, energetic inefficiency (leading to fatigue), and/or diminished performance.

Obviously, different types of athletes need different approaches to training. The optimal training program for a marathon runner is different from that of a hockey player; a powerlifter doesn't train the same way a sprinter does.

At the same time, the brain and nervous system play a key role for all athletes, regardless of their sport. For athletes who want to push the envelope of their physical capabilities, integrating a neurological approach into their training is essential.

This chapter covers the key components of a neurologically focused training program for strength athletes (we include Olympic weightlifters, powerlifters, and bodybuilders in this category), speed and power athletes (like sprinters and athletes competing in short duration track and field events), endurance athletes (such as marathon runners, cyclists, and triathletes), and team sport athletes.

Before going over the building blocks of optimal training in each athletic category, I want to lay out three neurological training principles that apply across the board: overtraining, specificity of adaptation, and the performance pyramid.

OVERTRAINING AND SPECIFICITY OF ADAPTATION

The principle of overtraining is simple: it's about pushing the body beyond past levels of performance so it can adapt to new levels of challenge.

If an athlete wants to improve, they actually need to create a deficit in the body—and do it consistently. Why? Creating a deficit in the body through overtraining changes their neurological programming.

Overtraining helps the brain understand that there's a survival benefit to adaptation. The brain responds to overtraining by supercompensating, or upgrading the body's systems and structures. In other words, instead of conserving resources in the short term, the brain sees that it's worth investing resources to increase the body's energy supply and build up strength in all the tissues being challenged through training—and it adapts accordingly.

WHAT DRIVES SPECIFICITY OF ADAPTATION? A COST-BENEFIT ANALYSIS IN THE BRAIN

Adaptations like building muscle, reorganizing neurological pathways, or forming a callus on the skin all require energy and raw materials. Because the body has a significant amount of work to do just to maintain itself, the brain will only invest additional energy and resources if it's clear that these investments are contributing to survival.

What drives the brain to invest and adapt in this way? It comes down to a straightforward cost-benefit analysis.

For example, if you lift a barbell one time and it irritates the skin on your hand, it won't be enough for the body to understand that it's worth investing resources toward laying down new skin proteins and building a callus.

On the other hand, if you lift a barbell three times a week for several months, then you cross a threshold. Because you're lifting the barbell consistently, the brain understands that channeling resources toward building that callus will be worth the investment—and yield more benefits than costs over time.

OVERTRAINING ON THE BELL CURVE

When we're working with individual athletes to improve performance, it's helpful to treat exercise the way doctors treat prescriptions. Before a doctor writes a prescription, they need to ensure that it's addressing the right problem (specificity)—and that it contains the right amount (dose).

Just as doctors can prescribe the wrong medicine for a particular health problem, coaches and clinicians can select the wrong exercises for a particular athlete.

On top of that, they can prescribe the wrong dose of exercise. Sometimes, they ask athletes to do too little, where they don't trigger any meaningful adaptations. Sometimes, they have them do too much, working out to the point where their form breaks down or where they can't maintain peak speed or strength.

In any training program, but especially when it comes to elite performance, there's an optimal amount of work, or exercise dosing, an athlete needs to do to gain maximum benefit from overtraining.

At NeuFit, when we're working to determine the optimal exercise dose for an athlete, we think in terms of a bell curve (Figure 7-1):

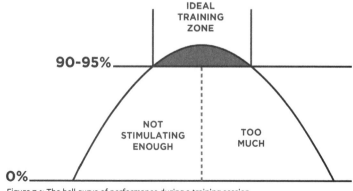

Figure 7-1: The bell curve of performance during a training session.

On this bell curve, the left side represents an athlete who trains too little to stimulate meaningful nervous system adaptations. (We sometimes call this a state of being "understimulated.") The right side shows an athlete who trains too much, working out past the point of excessive fatigue or breakdown—and opening the door to negative neurological adaptations that inhibit performance.

The peak of the bell curve represents the optimal amount of overtraining. This is the point where workouts create a deficit in the body that stimulates positive neurological and physiological adaptations. How do we determine an optimal amount of overtraining? I'll answer this question in the sections that follow.

THE DRAWBACKS OF TRAINING TOO HARD

While the drawbacks of training too little are clear, it's also important to understand why training too much is also counterproductive. It goes back to the concept of specificity of adaptation.

Once again, specificity is the idea that the body responds and adapts directly to its inputs and environment. How does this affect performance? If an athlete continues to train in a state of excessive fatigue where performance declines, the body will adapt to that level of diminished performance over time.

Imagine, for example, a soccer player doing a series of sprints with the goal of increasing their speed. When they reach the point of fatigue, their form breaks down, and they lose speed.

If they continue to sprint with poor form or reduced speed, this is exactly how their body will learn to move. There may be an adaptation in terms of endurance since their body will adjust to the specific demand of running at slower speeds for longer periods of time. Over time, however, the same drill designed to increase their speed can end up slowing them down.

HOW TO DETERMINE THE OPTIMAL LEVEL OF TRAINING

How do athletes know whether they're training too much or too little? How can they determine the optimal amount of training they need to support peak performance? There are two ways:

1. Measuring performance during training sessions
2. Monitoring the effects of training on health in the hours and days after a workout

During a training session, the key for any athlete is to maintain a certain level of performance. If they go below that performance threshold at any point during training, they need to rest until they can return to that level—or stop the session and start recovering.

For example, if an athlete is working on speed or power, we may want to use their vertical jump as a performance indicator during the session. If they can jump thirty inches, and we're trying to stay within a 10 percent range of overtraining, we would continue to retest their vertical jump and stop training if it dips below that 10 percent threshold (i.e., if they can't jump at least twenty-seven inches).

Besides measuring performance during training sessions, there are indicators of nervous system health that help us gauge whether an athlete is getting the right amount of training. Using these indicators to evaluate the body's response to workouts is a helpful tool to assess whether training is stimulating enough to trigger positive neurological adaptations. These indicators measure performance itself (i.e., whether performance improves throughout training) and the underlying health of the body (i.e., how well the body is meeting the demands of training and daily life).

If an athlete has low heart rate variability or suffers from frequent upper respiratory infections, for example, these are indicators that they're not recovering effectively from training. Most likely, they have too many stress hormones circulating in the body, which can lead to diminished performance and health problems over time. Poor sleep quality, digestive problems, and low energy are also indicators that the body is having trouble keeping up with the challenges of training.

In the next chapter, we'll examine these indicators of nervous system health in more detail. For now, it's important to understand that they can give us valuable information about the effectiveness of training.

THE PERFORMANCE PYRAMID

Though the specific components of an optimal training program vary from athlete to athlete, the building blocks of elite performance are basically the same.

At NeuFit, these building blocks form what we call the performance pyramid (Figure 7-2):

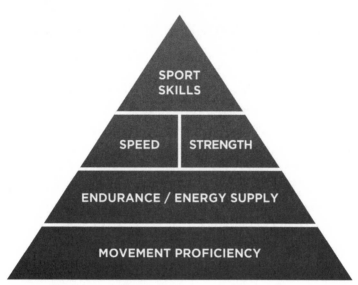

Figure 7-2: The performance pyramid.

At the base, or level one, of the pyramid is basic movement proficiency, which includes things like balanced muscle activation, proficiency in foundational movement patterns, and appropriate range of motion in all of the joints. Level two of the pyramid is endurance and energy systems (also known as "work capacity"), which includes having a healthy metabolic system to generate the energy needed for training and recovery. Strength and speed are at the third level. At the top of the pyramid are sport-specific skills.

Why do we approach performance training this way? The idea is that until athletes build a strong foundation in terms of movement, endurance, strength, and speed, their ability to improve their sport-specific skills will be limited.

In short, if an athlete goes straight to the top of the pyramid without laying the groundwork for their skills, the pyramid topples over. Sooner or later, their performance diminishes and/or they get injured.

Likewise, if an athlete only trains in one or two of the essential elements of performance, they not only reduce their chances of competing to the best of their ability, they also limit their chances of remaining competitive over time.

While it's important to work all the levels of the performance pyramid, the principle of specificity also dictates that different athletes need a different balance of these foundational components. In other words, we need to structure training so that it's relevant and appropriate to an athlete's sport.

The following sections explain how strength athletes, speed and power athletes, endurance athletes, and team sport athletes can apply the principles of the performance pyramid to compete at their absolute peak. We also cover some of the shifts that occur when we approach training from a neurological perspective.

THE PERFORMANCE PYRAMID FOR STRENGTH ATHLETES

For Olympic lifters, powerlifters, bodybuilders, and other strength athletes, there are a number of possible pitfalls when it comes to training. If we look at strength training in the context of the performance pyramid, some of the most common problems show up at the levels of basic movement proficiency and endurance.

As we've covered in previous chapters, basic movement proficiency involves things like movement coordination and joint mobility. Improving basic movement proficiency is often about correcting the body's software by changing the compensatory patterns the brain imposes on the body due to bad habits or previous injuries. Sometimes, we also need to address the body's hardware by loading the joints in absolute ranges of motion or using manual therapy techniques that remodel joint capsule tissue (the connective tissue that holds the joints together).

Strength athletes often have issues with basic movement proficiency when it comes to shoulder extension limitations during bench presses, for example, or ankle dorsiflexion and/or hip flexion during squats.

Why is basic movement proficiency important here? If an athlete has to round their back to make up for a lack of hip flexion, for instance, they increase the risk of injuring their spine.[60] Likewise, if a strength athlete can't get into a squat position without weight on their back—that is, if they need a weight to "push them into position"—it's a recipe for injury.

ENDURANCE TRAINING FOR STRENGTH ATHLETES

Besides basic movement proficiency, many strength athletes overlook endurance during their training. Olympic lifters and powerlifters, in particular, tend to assume endurance isn't important since they usually do only one to three reps at a time and have plenty of time to recover between lifts.

However, aerobic capacity is important for strength athletes, too. Why? In addition to improving general health,[61] it enhances their ability to recover between sets and workouts.[62]

By training themselves to recover more quickly between sets, strength athletes can fit in more quality work during each training session. And with a robust energy system to fuel more effective recovery between workouts, they can adapt more quickly and achieve strength gains faster than they would otherwise.

SPEED TRAINING FOR STRENGTH ATHLETES

Speed is another performance trait that strength athletes, especially powerlifters, often neglect in training. At NeuFit, we encourage strength athletes to engage in speed training because of its effect on coordination between opposing muscles (intermuscular coordination). Moving fast requires the opposing muscles to relax so they don't resist movement. Strength athletes can train to improve this type of coordination in two ways:

- Using lighter weights and moving with speed
- Engaging the muscles at every stage of movement during all lifts (If they're lifting weights, we want strength athletes to actively and intentionally pull the weight down and then push it up—instead of resisting the weight as it goes down.)

If someone is doing a bench press, for example, we instruct them to use their back muscles (e.g., lats, rhomboids) to actively pull the bar down and their front muscles (e.g., pectorals, front delts) to push it up. By using the back muscles as if they're actively performing a rowing or pulling movement, they create a neurological input of greater stability.

This feeling of greater stability reduces the perception of threat in the brain, which then triggers the brain to allow the greatest possible output in the front muscles as they press the weight back up. Plus, the enhanced coordination minimizes resistance in the back muscles as they press the weight up. (Pressing up the weight is challenging enough; athletes don't need any added resistance from inappropriate tension in opposing muscles.)

When strength athletes make a point of integrating traits like speed, endurance, and basic movement proficiency into their training routines, they do more than just reduce their risk of injury. By focusing on these traditionally overlooked areas in strength training, they can also gain a considerable edge when it comes to performance.

HOW THE PERFORMANCE PYRAMID CAN BENEFIT BODYBUILDERS

Like other strength athletes, bodybuilders spend the majority of their training time lifting weights and doing resistance-type exercises. However, they tend to focus more on building muscle mass than increasing strength.

Despite this difference, there are also significant benefits for bodybuilders who work at every level of the performance pyramid. Why? Like strength athletes, bodybuilders need a foundation of high-quality movement and joint mobility since they load their bodies with so much volume when they're lifting weights. Otherwise, they increase their risk of injury.

Endurance is another aspect of the performance pyramid that's important for bodybuilders since they need to be able to recover quickly within workouts in order to maximize the amount of work they put in during a session. They also need the energy to fuel the significant amount of protein synthesis and muscle growth that take place during recovery between workouts.

Strength and speed are also key aspects of performance for bodybuilders. The stronger they get, the more muscle fibers they recruit—and the more they stimulate their bodies to create new muscle tissue. The better their intermuscular coordination, the longer and harder they can train without getting injured or causing long-term damage.

Brad Rowe's experience speaks to how NeuFit and the performance pyramid can benefit bodybuilders. As a former NCAA Division I football player, Brad had endured his share of injuries and surgeries. After transitioning from football to professional bodybuilding, his injuries followed him.

Since he had to avoid overloading or re-injuring multiple parts of his body, his training was inconsistent. "I was often injured and in pain almost every day," he said. "To get through a workout, I usually had to take some kind of anti-inflammatory."

Brad started working with NeuFit after surgery on a torn bicep tendon. Though the doctors told him it would take sixteen weeks to heal, he recovered in about half that time: "Eight weeks after surgery, I was able to start training my bicep again," he said. "Fifteen weeks after surgery, I entered a bodybuilding competition and took third place."

After his recovery, Brad decided to use the Neubie in all of his training. Over time, the machine helped him drastically cut down on the amount of work he does at the gym. "What used to take me two to three hours now takes me about thirty minutes," he said.

In the meantime, he's able to train using lighter weights, focusing more of his attention on muscle activation through the entire range of motion. The result? He continues to build his movement proficiency and maintain his athleticism even as he trains for hypertrophy (muscle growth).

"This way," Brad said, "I don't have to sacrifice one aspect of my training while I work on another." What's more, he doesn't take anti-inflammatories or painkillers anymore—and he's rarely injured.

THE PERFORMANCE PYRAMID FOR SPEED AND POWER ATHLETES

To compete at the highest levels, it's also important for speed and power athletes to work at every level of the performance pyramid. In this section, we'll focus on sprinters, though the same principles apply to track and field and other athletes whose events require explosive movements. When it comes to these athletes, there are two main areas we focus on:

- Using plyometrics to achieve the optimal balance of velocity and strength
- Quantifying overtraining and avoiding submaximal training

INCREASED SPEED COMES FROM INCREASED POWER

Imagine a sprinter whose goal is to run a faster one hundred meter dash. Can running alone help them improve their time?

Not necessarily. If they're currently running one hundred meters in ten seconds, doing repeats at that same speed won't make them any faster. As highly regarded sports scientist Yuri Verkhoshanksy wrote:

"If the athlete repetitively performs the same sport exercise with the aim of executing it at the highest power output, his motor control system always uses the same engram [or archetype]...Because of this archetype, the athlete encounters great difficulty in changing the biodynamic structure of exercise when he repetitively strives to increase its power output."[63]

In other words, because of the specificity of adaptation, the athlete's body will respond by continuing to run at exactly the same speed.

So how can they run faster? To increase their speed, they need to increase their power, which is a combination of speed and strength. Where do they begin in terms of training? It depends on where they fall on the force-velocity curve.

The Force-Velocity Curve

The force-velocity curve (Figure 7-3) is an important frame of reference for speed and power athletes who want to improve their performance.

The principle behind the curve is simple. If an athlete has no load, they can move faster (as in the bottom right of the graph in Figure 7-3). Throwing something very light, like a baseball, is an example of an activity in this area of the force-velocity curve.

At the other extreme, if an athlete is bearing a heavy load, e.g., squatting or deadlifting a heavy weight, they can't move as quickly (as in the top left of the graph).

The goal of a sprinter, or any speed and power athlete, is to operate at the center of the force-velocity curve, where speed and strength meet. (Here, the load—which is the weight of their body without any external load or added weights—is in the middle of the curve.)

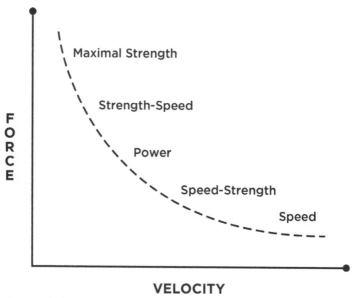

Figure 7-3: The force-velocity curve.

To optimize at this point of power, athletes need to challenge the nervous system with both greater load and greater velocity. Techniques like plyometrics are one of the most effective ways to work the nervous system at this level.

Plyometrics

Originally developed by Soviet scientists in the 1950s, plyometrics exercises are designed to increase power by inducing muscles to exert high levels of force in short amounts of time.[64] In other words, these exercises combine both speed and strength.

Using specialized jumping techniques, plyometrics train muscles to turn on quickly and transition quickly from eccentric to concentric contractions. In the process, the muscles grow capable of absorbing increasing amounts of force/load.

Why is the ability to absorb heavy loads important for speed and power athletes? With every stride, an elite sprinter has to support up to five times their body weight and generate that amount of force in a fraction of a second on a single leg.[65] For someone who weighs two hundred pounds, this could mean absorbing a thousand pounds of force on one leg with each stride.

It's impossible to train the body to absorb that magnitude of force by lifting weights in the gym. However, it is possible with plyometrics exercises. Most plyometric exercises involve repetitive jumps. The advantage of these reactive exercises is that they train the muscle-tendon complex to become more spring-like. And there are several good resources on how to perform them.[66]

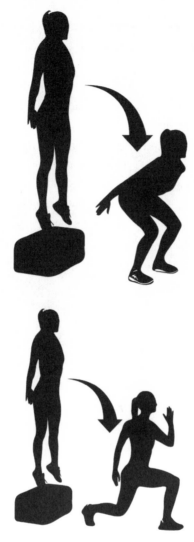

Figure 7-4: Plyometrics exercises include stepping off a ledge and landing in (a) a squat or (b) a lunge position.

In contrast to most traditional plyometrics programs, the NeuFit approach to plyometrics training devotes a large amount of time and effort to landings—like stepping or jumping off a ledge and landing in a squat or lunge position, as shown in Figure 7-4. Instead of moving quickly from landings to rebounding jumps, we've observed that having athletes spend more time on the landings themselves produces better results.

For example, when we spent a summer working with Greg, an NCAA Division I running back who wanted to increase his power, we focused primarily on landings as we gradually raised the height of his plyometrics jumps. Within weeks, his body was able to absorb heavier and heavier loads, and he progressed to jumping off a twelve-foot ledge and landing in a squat position wearing a weight vest. (Note: This training technique is risky and isn't designed for everybody. To minimize the risk of injury, athletes should only attempt these types of exercises under the supervision of a trained professional and with a significant amount of preparation.)

By the end of the summer, Greg reached the point where he could absorb approximately fifteen times its weight, or between 3,500 and 4,000 pounds of force. Increasing his power made a major difference in his speed as well as his performance: though already a powerful athlete, he was able to knock several tenths of a second off his forty-yard sprint and increase his vertical jump by over five inches.

QUANTIFYING OVERTRAINING AND AVOIDING SUBMAXIMAL TRAINING

From the point of view of neurological specificity, one of the most common pitfalls for speed and power athletes is submaximal training.

Submaximal training happens when athletes work out beyond the point where they can reach or maintain their peak level of speed. For example, if a one-hundred-meter sprinter continues to run intervals in a fatigued state, where they can only run at 85 percent capacity, for example, their body is adapting to moving at 85 percent capacity. What's more, if they keep on training in a state of fatigue, their form tends to break down, increasing their risk of injury.

To avoid falling into the submaximal training trap, it's important for speed and power athletes to work toward an optimal amount of overtraining (i.e., staying in that peak range on the bell curve in Figure 7-1). What does this involve?

The simplest approach to optimal overtraining for speed athletes is allowing enough time between sprints for them to recover completely—and stopping workouts when athletes can't get within 95 percent of their maximum speed. Though this might translate into fewer total reps initially, it ultimately helps athletes perform more reps at maximum speed.

In other words, proper overtraining emphasizes quality over quantity. Over time, thanks to the specificity of adaptation, performing more reps at maximum speed supports the body in learning to run faster.

BUILDING ENDURANCE AND MOVEMENT PROFICIENCY IN SPEED ATHLETES

Building endurance is another prerequisite for speed athletes looking to gain a considerable edge. As with other types of athletes, increased endurance helps them get more quality work done *within* training sessions by supporting their recovery between bouts of exercise.

Increased endurance can also help speed athletes recover

faster and more completely *between* training sessions. This allows them to lock in the positive adaptations from training and be ready to train again sooner since they're building robust energy systems that fuel and reinforce the body's recovery processes.

So how can speed athletes build endurance without sacrificing speed?

Instead of poor quality training—which includes things like repetitive, submaximal "wind sprints"—exercises like yielding isometrics and end range activations (ERAs) are some of the most effective endurance-building tools from a neurological perspective.

Yielding isometrics and ERAs (also covered in Chapter 6) build endurance while reinforcing proper mechanics. This has two advantages: minimizing the risk of injury and helping athletes avoid the flawed movement patterns and negative adaptations that often result from training while fatigued.

Without a slow-motion camera (or the eye of an experienced coach), it's difficult to detect breakdowns in mechanics while an athlete is sprinting. With yielding isometrics and ERAs, it's much easier to help athletes maintain and improve their quality of movement over time. When they perform these exercises in a controlled environment, we can easily see whether their positions are correct and when their form starts to break down. Along with plyometric-based landings, yielding isometrics and ERAs also help athletes achieve significant training effects in the eccentric domain.

ECCENTRIC MUSCLE CONTRACTIONS: AN IMPORTANT INJURY-PREVENTION TOOL

When the force applied to a muscle exceeds the force produced by the muscle itself, it induces what's known as an eccentric muscle contraction. As opposed to concentric muscle contractions, in which muscles shorten, eccentric muscle contractions happen when a muscle creates tension while it lengthens.

For example, if someone is doing a bicep curl, the lifting action is considered a concentric contraction of the bicep, whereas the lowering action is an eccentric contraction of the bicep.

Exercises that emphasize eccentric muscle contractions, such as the ERAs and yielding isometrics discussed above and in Chapter 6—as well as the plyometric landings like stepping off a box and landing in a squat or lunge—are especially helpful for preventing injury for all types of athletes. Why? Most non-contact sports injuries occur during the deceleration phase of movement when there's a high level of eccentric load on certain muscles (for example, in the quads while changing direction or cutting).[67]

In other words, the more an athlete trains their muscles to increase their eccentric capacity, the better equipped they are to handle high levels of force and quick changes of direction. In the process, they reduce their risk of getting injured.

THE PERFORMANCE PYRAMID FOR ENDURANCE ATHLETES

When training for a race, endurance athletes often focus on building stamina and not at all on improving strength and speed. While stamina obviously matters for these athletes, it's just as important for them to develop their strength, speed, and basic movement proficiency. Why?

The more strength an endurance athlete has in relation to their body weight, the more energy-efficient they can be. By improving their strength-to-weight ratio, these athletes can increase their stride length along with their capacity to propel themselves further with each step (or with each swim stroke in the pool or each pedal stroke on the bike)—all while using the same amount of energy.

ENERGY CAPACITY VERSUS ENERGY EFFICIENCY

Many endurance athletes invest significant time and energy trying to raise their VO_2 max, which is the maximum amount of oxygen the body can circulate to fuel the working muscles.

Why is VO_2 max important? If runner X has a VO_2 max of sixty liters per minute, for example, this means they can deliver sixty liters of oxygen to their muscles per minute while they're running. Meanwhile, if runner Y is the same weight as runner X and has a VO_2 max of 90 liters per minute, they can potentially create one-and-a-half times that amount of energy to fuel their activity.

Though increasing VO_2 max can improve performance for endurance athletes, I've observed that the benefits tend to be limited when focusing exclusively on endurance training and VO_2 max. Why? We're only as strong as our weakest link, and most endurance athletes have already developed their oxygen delivery systems, so they can only make relatively small, incremental improvements.[68]

Instead of focusing exclusively on VO_2 max training, I've found more opportunities to improve performance by focusing on improving overall energy efficiency (also known as local muscle endurance, or LME[69]). At NeuFit, we use the metaphor of a car to explain our training approach: if increasing VO_2 max is the equivalent of increasing the size of a gasoline car's engine, increasing overall energy efficiency is similar to improving the miles per gallon.

In other words, if we're working with a fixed amount of energy, how can we make the most of it? By increasing overall energy efficiency, we help runners channel as much energy as possible toward forward propulsion—and waste as little as possible on internal resistance.

The more a runner learns to relax their muscles, and the better their intermuscular coordination, the more energy-efficient they become. The results? Dramatically improved race times and dramatically fewer injuries, as Talaya's experience illustrates.

HOW THE PERFORMANCE PYRAMID HELPED AN ELITE MARATHONER ACHIEVE A PERSONAL BEST

As an elite long-distance runner, Talaya Frazier had already completed eight consecutive Boston marathons by the time she started training with NeuFit.

When she started training for her ninth Boston marathon, her schedule got even busier than usual. As time went by, it became more and more challenging to balance her training with her work for Cheyanna's Champions 4 Children (CC4C), the nonprofit organization she founded to help children in Texas with rare or undiagnosed conditions.

As her work with CC4C intensified, Talaya realized she could only put in half the time she usually did to prepare for the race. With these time limits in mind, we designed a training program for her that incorporated all the elements of the performance pyramid: strength, speed, and quality of movement, along with endurance and energy efficiency.

In the three months leading up to the marathon, Talaya cut her running mileage by about half. She substituted those miles with two to three NeuFit sessions per week.

In the end, she was amazed at the results. Taking a neurologically focused, energy-efficient approach to training not only helped her streamline her race preparations, it also helped her beat her personal best marathon time by several minutes and maintain her requalifying times for the next two years—with half the amount of training.

STRENGTH AND SPEED TRAINING FOR ENDURANCE ATHLETES

What does speed training for endurance athletes involve? Though the specifics vary from sport to sport, basic plyometrics exercises like the squat or lunge landings shown in Figure 7-4 are an effective speed-building tool.

Short sprint intervals are another useful speed-building exercise. For long-distance runners, in particular, workouts that include several six- to eight-second sprints with a full recovery in between are a good thing to incorporate into a training regimen. With these short sprints, endurance athletes improve their intermuscular coordination, which directly supports their energy efficiency.

Going back to the car metaphor, if a driver is hitting the brake and the accelerator at the same time, the car is going to waste energy trying to overcome the resistance from the brakes. In the case of endurance athletes, improving the coordination of opposing muscles is the equivalent of taking the foot off the brake to release the tension.

BASIC MOVEMENT PROFICIENCY FOR ENDURANCE ATHLETES

Chronic injuries are a common problem for many endurance athletes—as well as an indicator that something might be off-balance in their basic movement proficiency.

This is why having the right type and amount of joint mobility is so crucial for endurance athletes. Take a marathon runner like Talaya, who had been putting in dozens of miles a week. If something in her stride is off by even a fraction of an inch, that fraction of an inch gets compounded over tens of thousands of loading cycles. This can lead to irritation in various body tissues that can cause pain, stiffness, and eventually serious injury.

Though all the joints need mobility, we prioritize basic movement proficiency on the feet, ankles, knees, and hips for long-distance runners. When working with triathletes and/or swimmers, we pay particular attention to the shoulders.

The best way to assess whether an endurance athlete has the joint mobility they need for optimal performance is to work with a physical therapist or other trained professional. However, there are two simple self-assessments for joint mobility that can also be helpful: the deep squat and the ability to reach overhead. These two movement patterns date back tens of thousands of years. (Before modern toilets, we had to squat to defecate. And our earliest human ancestors used to hang from tree limbs.) Unfortunately, many modern humans are losing the ability to move their joints in these ways.

BREATHING, FATIGUE, AND ENDURANCE

Hand in hand with basic movement proficiency, breathing is another important consideration for endurance athletes. If a runner is hunched over, neglecting their form, and panting throughout a workout, they're basically training their body to enter and remain in a fight-or-flight state (as explained in Chapter 6). In the process, they're also triggering a fatigue response in the brain.

For endurance athletes, in particular, it's important to understand how fatigue works. Fatigue is actually a governor—a limiting influence—imposed by the brain. Again, since the brain is oriented first and foremost toward survival and protection, it automatically limits endurance or muscle output.

In an endurance context, the brain's main concern is that the body will run out of energy (or overheat) if athletes exert themselves too much or for too long. As a result, the brain reduces muscle output in order to conserve oxygen and energy, which results in fatigue.[70]

So how do endurance athletes keep fatigue from setting in? It starts with changing their neurological inputs, especially when it comes to breathing. As we covered in Chapter 6, the simple act of breathing through the nose, even during a hard workout, helps the nervous system handle greater levels of challenge while staying in a healthier, more parasympathetic state.

Breathing through the nose also helps counter the "respiratory muscle metaboreflex," a phenomenon that describes how increasing blood pressure and fatigue in the diaphragm reduce blood flow to the peripheral muscles.

Since performance tends to suffer when the breathing muscles themselves get fatigued, improving strength and endurance in the diaphragm can have a significant positive impact on performance. Practicing nose breathing during exercise is one of the best ways to strengthen the diaphragm, as is breathing against resistance (a.k.a inspiratory muscle training), which we'll cover in Chapter 9.[71]

In the meantime, it's important to understand that slowing down the breath rate and breathing from the diaphragm during intense training can actually change an athlete's neurological programming. When an athlete learns to slow their breathing at a point where they might have felt fatigued in the past, it sends a signal to the brain that they're not in a life-or-death situation. As a result, the brain doesn't try to limit or protect the body by sending out fatigue signals.

FROM REHAB TO ELITE PERFORMANCE: HOW NEUFIT HELPED A FLORIDA CLINIC EXPAND

NeuFit has really helped us in building our business around the Cross-Fit and/or Spartan Race type of athlete. And the Neubie has been an amazing catalyst to push us in the direction of these athletic, driven, high-performance individuals.

We've hired a strength and conditioning coach who also uses the Neubie on the performance side, so now we're able to expand our scope to serve patients all the way from the rehabilitation side through

THE PERFORMANCE PYRAMID FOR TEAM SPORT ATHLETES

Team sport athletes need a specific combination of movement proficiency, strength, speed, and endurance in addition to their sport-specific skills. The challenge is how to organize training in a way that builds all of these traits to support optimal performance.

More than any other type of athlete, team sport athletes need to invest significant time and effort into mastering skills related to their sport, including things like dribbling, shooting, and passing, along with strategy and tactics. What's the best way for these athletes to weave their skill work into their overall training plan, along with all the other levels of the performance pyramid?

For many team sport athletes, periodization is a framework that's often used to guide training. In its traditional form, periodization is a systematic approach to training planning designed to help athletes reach peak condition within a specific time frame.

One problem with the traditional periodization model is that it assumes all athletes respond the same way to the same training. However, there's a large body of research that shows this is not the case and that individual responses to the same training can vary widely.[72]

In light of the fact that one size does *not* fit all when it comes to periodization, we like to take a holistic approach at NeuFit. Looking at the body as an entire system, our approach to training integrates all four levels of the performance pyramid. It also involves continuously monitoring an athlete's response to training, using the indicators of nervous system health and readiness outlined in the next chapter.

Approaches to periodization, or deciding when to work on different parts of the performance pyramid, vary depending on the level and development of an athlete. For beginners, a "parallel" model of periodization, in which they train simultaneously in multiple areas, is often the best approach. Why? Beginners are generally more responsive to training and can shift more easily between the different attributes of performance.

As athletes grow more advanced, they need more significant stimuli to improve performance in a particular area. For advanced or professional athletes, a "serial" or "block" approach to periodization, in which training focuses on individual attributes of performance, is usually more effective.[73]

How does this look in practice? Sometimes, it involves a two- to four-week block in which athletes concentrate on strength, endurance, or speed, paying minimal attention to other aspects of performance.

Even if we adjust periodization training to fit an individual athlete's needs, we need to keep in mind that both "parallel" and "block" approaches are designed for athletes training for a specific event, like a track meet or a powerlifting competition.

These periodization strategies don't necessarily make sense

for a professional hockey player like Brent Burns, who has to perform at an elite level over an eighty-two-game season. In Brent's case, and for other athletes competing at his level, it's impossible to implement a "block" periodization strategy during the season because he can't pause to focus on a single aspect of his performance. (Though it's possible to do it in the off-season.) Instead, it's crucial for him to work systematically to maintain (or even improve) all the key areas of performance at all times.

Most—but not all—of Brent's endurance, speed, strength, and skill work is naturally incorporated into practices and games. For him and for other athletes in his position, a big part of successfully navigating a long season involves balancing recovery and accumulated fatigue from practices, games, and travel (and all the sleep and nutrition challenges that come with travel) with additional training.

"Everybody's goal at the start of the year is to play every game," he said. "But there's a lot of work that goes into making that happen. Your body can maintain its hockey playing, you think. But your strength levels and everything else just deteriorate through the year."

After games, for example, team sport athletes like Brent experience fatigue and reductions in performance depending on their playing time, the amount of physical contact, and other factors.[74] These deficits can sometimes last from forty-eight to seventy-two hours.[75]

To ease the wear and tear on his body between games, Brent used the Neubie to stimulate the vagus nerve, which helped increase his parasympathetic nervous system activity, accelerate his recovery, and restore his baseline function.

In addition, he was able to incorporate quick (fifteen- to thirty-minute) training sessions with the Neubie to keep his strength, speed, mobility, and endurance at peak levels throughout the season. Toward the end of the season, when the cumulative effects of fatigue and injury typically slow down most NHL players, his body still felt fresh, "like it had in my first few seasons."

Throughout the season, Brent also learned to use a series of indicators to monitor the health of his nervous system and further improve his performance. These indicators—which played a key role in helping him decide when to train and when to recover—are the subject of the next chapter.

PART 3

THE NEUFIT METHOD FOR SUSTAINABLE NEUROLOGICAL HEALTH

8

HOW TO ASSESS NERVOUS SYSTEM HEALTH: THE PRIMARY INDICATORS

After walking away from competitive bodybuilding, Diego ran into a series of health issues. Besides hormonal imbalances and serious skin problems, he was also dealing with chronic high blood pressure, though he was just thirty-seven years old.

By the time he started training with NeuFit, he'd already been taking beta-blockers—a blood pressure-reducing medication that curbs sympathetic nervous system activity in the heart and blood vessels—for a few years.

"The beta-blockers were keeping my blood pressure under control," he said. "But whenever I exercised, I could feel my body putting on the brakes." By restraining his body's stress response, the medication kept him from raising his heart rate enough to push himself in his workouts and stimulate the nervous system in any meaningful way.

During our initial sessions with Diego, we identified the areas of his body where his nervous system was restricting activity and movement—then we worked to reset them. To improve parasympathetic nervous system function, we focused on proper breathing, teaching him to slow his breath rate and breathe through his nose during workouts.

We also used the Neubie to directly stimulate the vagus nerve—one of the most powerful nerve bundles in the body—to further strengthen his parasympathetic nervous system.

"Within three weeks of starting the training with NeuFit," Diego said, "my resting heart rate decreased by twenty beats per minute. My blood pressure returned to a normal range. But the biggest thing was I stopped taking beta-blockers. And I haven't taken them since." (Note: Diego stopped taking his medication under the supervision of his doctor. Anyone considering making changes to their prescription medication should consult their doctor first.)

THE VARIOUS INDICATORS OF NERVOUS SYSTEM HEALTH

In Diego's case, high blood pressure was the most obvious sign that his nervous system was functioning at a less than optimal level. Along with high blood pressure and other chronic lifestyle-related diseases, there are a series of additional indicators that can give us important clues about the health of the nervous system.

Besides providing a window into nervous system function, these indicators are valuable tools for monitoring the effectiveness of training, as well as assessing overall fitness and health.

In this chapter, we'll focus on how to use the following indicators to evaluate nervous system health:

- Heart rate variability
- Heart rate response to training
- Energy levels and libido
- Mental acuity
- Sleep quality
- Appetite
- Body composition
- Bowel function
- Immune function
- Blood pressure and chronic lifestyle-related diseases

ESTABLISHING A BASELINE

The rehab and fitness methods featured in Parts 1 and 2 of this book directly address the nervous system—so they tend to have a significant positive impact on the indicators of nervous system health. In other words, taking a neurologically focused approach to rehab and training usually leads to improvements in brain and nervous system function.

Some of these improvements show up quickly, almost in real time, while others take longer to manifest. Heart-rate variability, sleep, sex drive, and appetite, for example, can change from day to day. However, things like chronic high blood pressure, as well as lifestyle-related diseases like diabetes, are conditions that develop over time and also take time to improve.

Given the range of possible responses to rehab and training, it's important to establish a baseline. By noting each person's starting point when it comes to things like heart rate variability, sleep quality, and digestive function, we can clearly assess the effects of rehab and training on their nervous system over time—and adjust our approach whenever we need to.

THE INDICATORS ARE INTERCONNECTED

Since all of these indicators are tied to the nervous system, they're all interrelated. If someone is spending most of their time in a sympathetic-dominant state, there are generally multiple signs, like high blood pressure, poor sleep quality, and low heart rate variability. But if someone stays in a parasympathetic state for too long, never challenging themselves through exercise or in other ways, long-term health and performance will suffer, too. Ultimately, it comes down to balance. To find that balance, we need to see the overall picture.

This is why it's important to evaluate the indicators of nervous system function collectively rather than individually. Instead of drawing conclusions or making decisions based on a single indicator, we want to consider them as a whole in the context of rehab, fitness training, and long-term health.

HEART RATE VARIABILITY: A KEY INDICATOR OF NERVOUS SYSTEM HEALTH

Heart rate variability is one of the most powerful indicators of nervous system health. But what exactly is heart rate variability, and why is it important?

Heart rate variability is a measure of the time interval between heartbeats in milliseconds.[76] As with bodily functions like breathing, digestion, and elimination, heart rate variability is controlled by the autonomic nervous system.

HEART RATE VARIABILITY AND THE AUTONOMIC NERVOUS SYSTEM

The autonomic nervous system, also known as the automatic nervous system, includes both the sympathetic and parasympathetic nervous systems. On any given day, the body moves along a continuum between these two sides of the nervous system.

As I wrote in Chapter 6, optimal nervous system function is characterized by the ability to shift between states of high (sympathetic) activity and recovery (parasympathetic) as often as necessary. Over time, if the body gets locked in any one state for too long, problems arise, from blood pressure and blood sugar issues to neurological and digestive disorders.

So how do we know when the body is spending too much time on either side of the nervous system? One of the best ways is to track heart rate variability.

Since it's controlled by the autonomic nervous system, heart rate variability is a powerful tool to measure the balance of that system. Essentially, it's a snapshot of how the autonomic nervous system is functioning at a particular moment in time.

OPTIMAL HEART RATE VARIABILITY

High heart rate variability is generally a sign of healthy nervous system function since it indicates that the body can move easily along the continuum between the sympathetic and parasympathetic nervous systems.

How high should it be? To understand what's behind optimal heart rate variability, let's look at a hypothetical example:

Imagine patient X's resting heart rate is sixty beats per minute, and they average exactly one second between heartbeats. If this is the case, they have zero heart rate variability because the time interval between each heartbeat is exactly the same. This is an indicator of suboptimal nervous system function.

By contrast, healthy heart rate variability looks like this: a few beats with a slightly longer interval in between, say 1.1 seconds, and a few beats with a slightly shorter time interval in between, say .9 seconds.

In this case, the interval between heartbeats varies up from the average by 0.1 seconds and down from the average by 0.1 seconds. The heart rate goes as low as fifty-four beats per minute and as high as sixty-six beats per minute while still averaging sixty beats per minute. This might not sound like a significant variation, but it's a reasonably high value in terms of heart rate variability metrics.

OTHER FACTORS AFFECT HEART RATE VARIABILITY

While higher heart rate variability is generally a sign of better nervous system health, it's important to keep in mind that it can differ substantially from one person to the next. Factors like age, gender, lifestyle, and fitness level have an influence, so it's important to take them into account when determining an optimal amount of heart rate variability for each person.

Instead of focusing on what's "normal" or "right," at NeuFit, we prefer to use both individual measurements and population norms when monitoring heart rate variability. For example, if someone's baseline measurement of seventy-five milliseconds is better than 80 percent of the population in their age group, it gives us a good frame of reference. However, we still want to observe how their heart rate variability increases or decreases over time in the context of their training and lifestyle choices.

HOW TO MEASURE HEART RATE VARIABILITY

There are many different devices that measure heart rate variability, along with different software programs that calculate a standard deviation and plug that into a variety of formulas to come up with a value for heart rate variability.[77]

Since it's difficult to make these calculations manually, I recommend wearable devices to monitor heart rate variability on a daily basis.

Based on my experience, the two wearable devices I prefer are the Biostrap and the Oura Ring. I like them for three reasons:

- They're easy to wear (one is a ring and one a wrist strap).
- They're accurate and consistent. In fact, both devices are clinically validated,[78] and both were used as part of the NIH (National Institutes of Health) studies looking at biometrics to predict COVID diagnoses.[79]
- They measure heart rate variability during sleep.

Why is it important to measure heart rate variability during sleep? During sleep, we don't consciously control our breathing or other bodily activities, so these devices typically provide unbiased readings that are a relatively accurate reflection of the actual status of the body. Besides measuring heart rate variability, they also grade the body's overall current functional capacity and neurological responses to stress and challenge. (Note: If you already own a FitBit, Whoop, Garmin, or similar wearable device, you can also use it to track these indicators during sleep.)

In addition to wearable devices, some doctors and therapists invest in high-end clinical devices to measure heart rate variability, including EKGs, chest straps, or wrist cuffs with electrodes. These devices are also valuable measurement tools, particularly when monitoring changes before and after an exercise session or evaluating someone's level of readiness for a workout.

HOW THE NEUBIE CAN IMPACT HEART RATE VARIABILITY: A CLINICIAN WEIGHS IN

We almost found out by accident how much the Neubie affects the autonomic nervous system based on heart rate variability. Previously, we'd been using a fingertip heart rate variability tracking device. The first year we used the Neubie, I noticed patients almost always saw an increase in heart rate variability. It was always higher after using the Neubie and to a much greater degree than with anything we had seen in previous years.

Recently, we decided to invest in an advanced diagnostic heart rate variability system and have our DPT (Doctor of Physical Therapy) interns study the results as part of their research. We looked at 600 patients and found two very clear patterns:

- *An intense Neubie treatment or training session caused heart rate variability to dip that day because the body was intentionally*

that it's possible, not to mention safe and beneficial, for highly trained athletes to go beyond traditional estimates for maximum heart rate. For example, imagine an elite athlete whose heart rate is around 100 beats per minute in a state of moderate activity or recovery between exercises. If they break into a full sprint, they can raise their heart rate above 200 beats per minute—well above the prescribed maximum—and have no problems recovering afterward.

This level of heart rate response isn't limited to elite athletes, however. As long as their nervous systems are healthy and functioning well, people of all ages and abilities are physiologically capable of going beyond conventional estimates when it comes to heart rate and heart rate response. (At the same time, it's important to keep in mind that pushing anyone to their maximum heart rate has inherent risks. Before practicing any type of rigorous cardiovascular exercise, people need to get clearance from their doctors.)

To measure heart rate response to exercise, we use chest strap or arm band heart rate monitors, which are more sensitive than the typical heart monitor. I like the Biostrap interface here, using the chest strap or arm band instead of the wrist strap designed for tracking during sleep. (Other options on the market can work, but I don't recommend using a regular wrist strap or a watch in this case. It takes specialized technology to respond quickly enough to measure these types of heart rate responses.)

BLOOD PRESSURE

Just as the heart responds when someone starts to train or be physically active, so should the blood pressure. In a healthy nervous system, blood pressure increases in parallel with the heart rate.

Measuring someone's heartbeat and taking their blood pressure during a workout is a good way to gauge whether the two are increasing in tandem. If they're not, it's another sign that the nervous system is compromised and that the brain may be imposing limits on the body.

Since the same neurological mechanisms are responsible for regulating blood pressure and heart rate variability, these two variables often correlate with one another. In other words, differences or improvements in heart rate variability usually precede or happen along with improvements in blood pressure. This was the case with Diego, whose story started this chapter: as his heart rate variability went up, his blood pressure began to trend into a healthy range.

AN OPTIMAL LEVEL OF BLOOD PRESSURE

When it comes to blood pressure, as with all of the indicators of nervous system health, the goal is an optimal level, which is neither too high nor too low. For most people, this level is around 120 over seventy at rest.

Though high blood pressure—a result of too much sympathetic nervous system activity—is a well-known health issue, low blood pressure can also be a problem. For some people, low blood pressure—specifically low diastolic blood pressure, which measures the ability of the arteries to maintain their structural integrity between heartbeats—may be a sign that they've become depleted from spending too much time in fight-or-flight mode and have fallen into in a parasympathetic-dominant "freeze" state.

According to multiple studies focusing on blood pressure among older adults,[81] low diastolic blood pressure in elderly people is often a good predictor of mortality. Researchers found that people with comparatively low diastolic blood pressure demonstrated greater frailty, more fatigue, and lower energy levels than their peers.

ENERGY LEVELS AND NERVOUS SYSTEM HEALTH

We all want to have enough energy to perform our daily activities. So at what point does a lack of energy become a cause for concern? Since energy levels are relative and vary widely from person to person, it's difficult to measure them objectively.

Yet, it's still possible to evaluate energy levels in the context of nervous system health. At NeuFit, we make these evaluations based on clients' responses to these questions about their daily habits and behaviors:

- Do you have enough energy to accomplish everything you want to on a given day?
- Are you able to stay present and focused as you go through your daily activities?
- Do you struggle to stay awake during the day? Do you need caffeine or a sugary snack to perk up in the afternoon?
- During an afternoon lull, is a ten- to twenty-minute nap, a quick meditation, or a walk outside enough to reinvigorate you and give you the energy to take on the rest of the day?

A client's responses to these questions can tell us whether their energy level is lower than it should be. If they struggle to focus, frequently feel fatigued, and/or rely on stimulants to make it through the day, then it's important to take a close look at the training, environmental, and lifestyle factors that might be contributing to their lack of energy. (In the next chapter, we'll cover these lifestyle factors in detail.)

MENTAL ACUITY AND THE NERVOUS SYSTEM

Mental acuity goes hand in hand with energy level as far as being an indicator of nervous system health. When the nervous system is functioning well, we have the mental energy and focus to work deeply. If our underlying physiology isn't operating at its peak, then the quality of our work and thought processes tend to suffer.

Only after the brain has fulfilled its so-called lower functions is it able to channel energy toward things like executive and cognitive function. To put it another way, if all of the brain's energy is going toward immediate survival and protection, there isn't enough left over for higher-level cognitive processes.

Research demonstrates that the body's energy and fatigue status can affect attention,[83] academic performance,[84] and decision-making[85] (and this applies to judges[86] and doctors[87] as well). Ultimately, if we can't think clearly, solve problems, access memory, or make intelligent decisions, then it's usually a sign that there's an imbalance in the brain and nervous system.

NEUFIT RECOMMENDATIONS FOR TESTING OTHER ASPECTS OF BRAIN FUNCTION

Besides monitoring mental acuity, we also test brain functions like processing speed and reaction time over the course of rehab and training at NeuFit. Why? These brain functions are yet another way for us to assess neurological health as well as observe changes in the nervous system.

Here are some of the tools we use:

The ten-second finger tapping test is one of the best techniques for assessing the speed of neurological transmission. This test works the way it sounds: a smartphone app measures how many times a person can tap on their screen in ten seconds. Besides measuring neurological transmission speed, it's also a helpful tool for assessing the speed of processing and coordination. With many clients, we see these test results improve over time. This is significant since tapping tests like this are connected with maintaining myelination and brain processing speed over the course of a lifetime.[88]

Brain Gauge and **WAVi** are software programs that deliver useful cognitive assessments. Both show changes over time that indicate improved or diminished neurological function, and both measure brain processing speed. While WAVi is designed for clinicians, Brain Gauge is more accessible for home users.

SLEEP AND THE NERVOUS SYSTEM

In addition to the indicators of neurological health we've covered so far, sleep quality and sleep quantity reveal a great deal about the function of the nervous system. Generally speaking, sleep quality is at least as important—and sometimes more important—than sleep quantity in terms of its impact on overall health and the nervous system. In the sections that follow, we'll cover the components of sleep quality. In the next chapter, we'll look at strategies for improving sleep.

SLEEP QUALITY

High-quality sleep includes two main phases: deep sleep and rapid eye movement (REM) sleep. Each of these phases serves a different but equally important neurological purpose.

During deep sleep, which usually takes place during the first half of the night, the body is primarily involved in processes of replenishment and physical repair, rebuilding the muscles, bones, and connective tissue.

These processes include replenishing energy in the brain[89] and clearing out the glymphatic system (the lymphatic circulation system that removes metabolic waste buildup from the brain).[90] In the absence of this glymphatic clearing process, amyloid plaques build up in the brain, potentially leading to neurological diseases like Alzheimer's and dementia. This is one of the reasons deep sleep is vital for neurological health.

By and large, people enter the REM phase after deep sleep, with more REM taking place during the second half of the night. Since the brain is more active during REM sleep, it's characterized by intense dreams. During REM sleep, the brain makes new connections, consolidates memories, and/ or moves memories from short-term to long-term memory. Essentially, REM sleep is when neurological reorganizing takes place.

Interestingly, research shows[91] that REM sleep tends to increase during periods of intense learning. When the brain learns new mental or physical skills that demand high levels of coordination and concentration, people need more REM sleep to integrate this new information. Throughout this book, we've focused on the importance of neurological adaptations: REM sleep is when they actually happen.

SLEEP QUANTITY

The ideal quantity of sleep varies from person to person. It's also a byproduct of what happens during the day. The harder someone trains, the more deep sleep they typically need to repair the body.[92] At the same time, people who lead sedentary or unhealthy lifestyles often have high levels of inflammation and other general health problems, so they often need more sleep to recover and repair.

In terms of nervous system health, the more time a person spends in deep and REM sleep, the better—even if they get fewer total hours of sleep.

Take person X, who stays in bed for six hours and spends over 50 percent of that time between deep and REM sleep. Compare them to person Y, who spends eight hours in bed but only 20 percent of that time in deep and REM sleep. Even though person X is spending less time in bed overall, their relatively high ratio of restorative sleep is more beneficial for the nervous system and overall health.

On average, the sleep ratio for adults includes 10 to 25 percent deep sleep and 10 to 25 percent REM sleep.[93] Lighter stages of sleep make up the remainder of the time. Though restful, these lighter stages aren't as significant when it comes to repair, regeneration, and nervous system function.

From a neurological perspective, a good target for a night of high-quality sleep consists of 50 percent of the night shared between deep and REM sleep. However, the ratios between deep and REM sleep can fluctuate.

MEASURING SLEEP QUALITY

In terms of measuring sleep quality, sleep studies—which usually involve participants sleeping with electrodes on their heads to measure their brainwaves throughout the night—are the gold standard.

In the absence of sleep studies, the Oura Ring, one of the wearable devices I mentioned earlier in this chapter, is a great tool for tracking sleep (in addition to heart rate variability and other indicators of nervous system health). The Oura Ring monitors the amount of time spent in light sleep versus deep and REM sleep.[94] And I speak from personal experience when I say that having access to these objective measurements is important since it helps us evaluate sleep in the context of nervous system health over time.

Every morning, the Oura gives me a readout like the one shown in Figure 8-1, which is a screenshot from my phone. I chose to share this readout because it's an example of high-quality sleep. On this particular night, I had 44 percent deep sleep and 32 percent REM sleep, meaning I spent 76 percent of the night between the two most impactful stages of sleep.

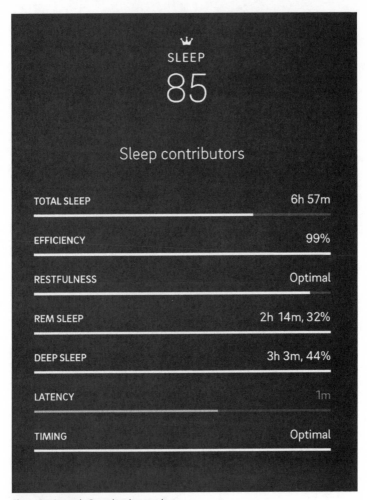

Figure 8-1: A sample Oura ring sleep readout.

Since its algorithm weighs sleep quantity over sleep quality—and my total sleep on this particular night was just under seven hours—the Oura ring only gave me an 85 percent sleep score. But given the large percentage of high-quality sleep, I would argue that this was an efficient night of sleep. These types of nights have become increasingly common for me as I've applied the neurologically focused training and lifestyle strategies covered in these pages. In fact, improving the efficiency of my sleep often allows me to fit in an extra hour or two of focused work before my kids wake up in the morning—which is how I was able to write this book.

Besides readouts from wearable devices like the Oura ring, snoring is another valuable measurement of sleep quality. If the nervous system is functioning well and the body is healthy overall, a person shouldn't snore. If someone snores frequently, it can be a sign of inflammation in the throat and other areas of the body, mouth breathing, and/or sleep apnea (when someone stops breathing for brief periods during sleep, which is disruptive and reduces sleep quality).

Waking up feeling rested, refreshed, and ready for the day ahead is another way to gauge sleep quality. Though objective measurements are important and valuable, the subjective experience of feeling good at the beginning of the day is worth considering as an indicator, too.

APPETITE AND THE NERVOUS SYSTEM

Since blood sugar is intimately connected to the presence of stress hormones, blood sugar levels and appetite also give us important clues about overall health and the health of the nervous system.

To understand the impact of blood sugar levels on the body, let's look at an example of a sedentary person who eats high-glycemic foods that spike their blood sugar. These blood sugar spikes trigger the release of insulin, which leads to blood sugar absorption in the tissues of the muscles, liver, and/or fat cells. Ultimately, large quantities of insulin cause blood sugar to drop, triggering the appetite.

Unfortunately, this scenario is all too common today. Instead of eating when their bodies need nutrients, many people feel the urge to eat every two or three hours because their blood sugar is going up and down like a roller coaster. The result? They consume too many poor-quality calories, which can lead to problems like obesity, inflammation, and other long-term health issues.

When people can comfortably go for longer periods of time between meals, say five or more hours, it's a sign that their blood sugar is stable. It's also indicative of metabolic flexibility, a healthy state where the body is capable of drawing on both fat and carbohydrates for fuel, pulling energy from whatever source is available.[95]

Besides indicating stable blood sugar and metabolic flexibility, going for longer periods between meals allows energy that would normally go toward digestion—which demands an enormous amount of the body's resources—to be used for repair and regeneration.

However, going for long periods between meals may not be the best approach for people who are training hard, trying to gain mass, and/or working to repair an injury since they often require extra calories and have an increased appetite. In these cases, increased hunger can be a sign that someone is training effectively. Since their body needs additional nutrients for effective recovery and regeneration, the brain triggering a feeling of hunger is an indicator that it's shifting into "rest-and-digest" mode, preparing to take in nutrients and put them to use during the recovery process.

On the other hand, if something is off balance in training

or rehab, we sometimes see a decrease in appetite due to excessive sympathetic nervous system activity. Because stress hormones mobilize energy, the body perceives that there's enough energy available in the blood and suppresses feelings of hunger.

How do we determine whether appetite patterns are in line with optimal nervous system function? By observing them in relation to the other indicators of nervous system health described in this chapter, including heart rate variability, body composition, and bowel function.

If the other indicators suggest that the nervous system is working well, then it's safe to assume that a "healthy appetite" is actually healthy. If the indicators are off, then increased appetite can be a sign of blood sugar dysregulation and other metabolic issues that ultimately impact—and are impacted by—the nervous system.

BODY COMPOSITION AND THE NERVOUS SYSTEM

In previous chapters, we explored some of the dangers and consequences of having excessive amounts of stress hormones in the body, i.e., spending too much time in a sympathetic-dominant state.

Yet another downside of being in fight-or-flight mode for too long is its effect on body composition. When dealing with high levels of stress hormones, the body basically breaks down muscle and stores fat—the exact opposite of what most people want.[96]

This is why body composition—which describes the ratio of

fat, bone, water, and muscle in the body—is another meaningful indicator of nervous system health.

IDEAL BODY COMPOSITION

What does ideal body composition look like? It varies according to gender and activity levels.[97] For the average man who wants to stay fit and healthy, the ideal body fat percentage is typically around 10 to 15 percent. Anything lower than that usually requires significant effort and strict dieting.

For some elite athletes, 8 to 10 percent body fat is sustainable. Others, especially bodybuilders, train to the point where their body fat is between 5 and 6 percent. However, this low body fat percentage isn't sustainable for most people, especially since the brain and bodily organs need fat in order to function. (In the next chapter, we'll explore this topic in more detail.)

For women, a healthy target in terms of body composition is 14 to 22 percent body fat. With high levels of exercise, women may get down to the 10 to 13 percent range, but any lower than that typically isn't sustainable.

Should body composition change as people age? Though people often carry more fat as they grow older, this is more of a function of their lifestyles than the passage of time. As people age, it's natural and acceptable for their body fat to increase by a percent or two, but significant increases in body fat generally aren't good for health.

That said, the goal isn't to stay thin with age. In terms of longevity and body composition, we want to help people develop strength and maintain muscle mass—not to stay (or grow) thin.

Ultimately, it's better to be stronger and carry some extra body fat than to be thin and weak, particularly as people grow older. In fact, many studies show that increased muscle mass and muscle strength can help people live longer.[98]

HOW TO MEASURE BODY COMPOSITION

Bioelectrical impedance analysis devices, also known as body fat scales, send a mild electrical current through the body to determine body fat percentage and muscle mass. They're a popular, accessible way to measure body composition. DEXA scans, which use x-rays, are the gold standard for accuracy. However, medical professionals have to perform them, and they're less widely available. Some people also utilize hand-held calipers to measure skinfold, which is less expensive but can be fairly accurate with an experienced user. (However, it's important to keep in mind that calipers only measure body fat—not muscle mass, water, or bone density.)

As useful as these tools are, we don't necessarily need sophisticated tests to measure body composition. Sometimes, it's enough to look in the mirror and see whether the body looks toned and muscular or soft and pudgy.

BOWEL FUNCTION AND THE NERVOUS SYSTEM

Along with appetite, body composition, and the other indicators in this chapter, bowel function is a vital tool for assessing nervous system health. How exactly does bowel function relate to the nervous system?

For one thing, the digestive organs are innervated, or stimulated, by the vagus nerve, a major parasympathetic nervous system pathway that runs from the brainstem to the colon. The vagus nerve stimulates peristalsis, the pumping action of the digestive tract. In short, the brain and nervous system are responsible for regulating much of what happens in the gut.

Given this link between the brain and the bowels, it naturally follows that observing gut function can give us valuable information about nervous system function.

In fact, based on my clinical experience, I would argue that the most direct path to improving bowel function goes through the nervous system. Though fiber and probiotics can be helpful when it comes to dealing with digestive problems, we also need to recognize the influence of the brain and nervous system on digestive health.[99]

When working with clients at NeuFit, we often see how nervous-system-focused activities and treatments—like intentional breathing practices or the Neubie's "Master Reset" (more on this in the next chapter)—help trigger bowel movements or improve regularity in cases of constipation.

THE NEUROLOGY OF A GUT FEELING

Neurological signals that travel from the brain to the bowels play a key role in regulating digestion and overall bowel function. However, the information that travels from the gut to the brain is just as important.

In fact, there are more sensory fibers along the nerve pathways that travel from the gut to the brain than vice versa. That is, the brain is constantly receiving an enormous amount of information from the bowels.

That "gut feeling" often described as intuition? It literally comes from the gut. This is part of the reason why gut health is so important for brain health.[100]

ASSESSING GUT HEALTH

In terms of nervous system health, what do we need to look for when evaluating bowel function?

There are two main factors:

- Bowel transit time, or how long it takes the body to go from eating to elimination
- The color, consistency, and smell of the stool

When it comes to bowel transit time—the time between when we ingest food and when it shows up in the stool—approximately twenty-four hours is ideal. We can test transit time by eating something we can actually see in the stool, like corn or beets. Sometimes, medical professionals use food coloring or other dyes.

In terms of stool color and consistency, the easiest way to assess them is to compare them with the samples on the Bristol Stool Chart (Figure 8-2), which provides insights into the composition of gut bacteria[101] and serves as a high-quality measure of transit time.[102]

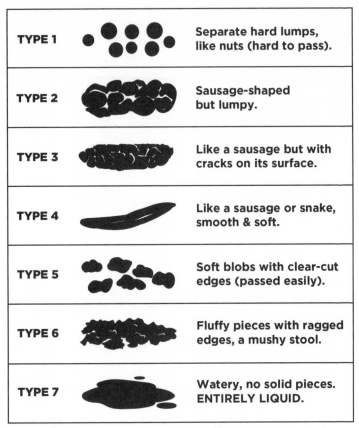

TYPE 1		Separate hard lumps, like nuts (hard to pass).
TYPE 2		Sausage-shaped but lumpy.
TYPE 3		Like a sausage but with cracks on its surface.
TYPE 4		Like a sausage or snake, smooth & soft.
TYPE 5		Soft blobs with clear-cut edges (passed easily).
TYPE 6		Fluffy pieces with ragged edges, a mushy stool.
TYPE 7		Watery, no solid pieces. ENTIRELY LIQUID.

Figure 8-2: The Bristol stool chart for analyzing bowel movements.

On this chart, Type 1 represents stool with a long transit time, say two or more days.[103] Since it's spent so much time in the intestines, most of the water from the fecal matter gets absorbed, so it exits the body in the form of tiny, dry balls. This type of stool can be a sign of sluggish bowels or blockages related to constipation.

In terms of nervous system health, Type 1 stool is also a sign of deficient parasympathetic nervous system activity. In other words, it can be an indicator that the body is spending too much time in a sympathetic/fight-or-flight state and not enough time in rest-and-digest mode.

At the other end of the spectrum, mushy stool and diarrhea, Types 6 and 7 on the Bristol Stool Chart, are usually signs that the body can't process healthy food and that the bowels are irritated. In this case, bowel transit time is too short. As a result, the small intestines don't have a chance to extract valuable nutrients, and/or the large intestine can't absorb the water the body needs.

Sometimes, Types 6 and 7 stool can indicate mild to severe food poisoning. In this case, diarrhea is a positive adaptation or a sign that the body is taking action to get rid of toxins instead of absorbing harmful substances and bacteria. If it's temporary, diarrhea isn't something we want to stop. However, if it goes on for a period of time, then there's an imbalance we need to address—at least part of which is at the level of the nervous system.

WHAT DOES IDEAL BOWEL FUNCTION LOOK LIKE?

Type 4 on the Bristol Stool Chart is what we consider optimal. In this case, the consistency of the stool is smooth but not liquid, meaning that enough water has been absorbed to make it solid yet soft enough to pass with ease.

Optimal, Type 4 stool doesn't stick to the toilet bowl or to the backside. (If it does, it's probably also sticking to the inside of the colon.) That is, there's no need to do much wiping since there's little to no fecal matter left along the rectal walls after a healthy bowel movement.

Besides the appearance and texture of the stool, frequency is another factor to consider when it comes to optimal bowel function. Ideally, we should have a bowel movement after every meal. This is what happens in nature, after all.

The majority of animals, along with indigenous populations who live in close contact with the natural world, move their bowels shortly after eating.[104] The fact that this doesn't happen for most of us (as few as three bowel movements per week are still considered "normal" in modern society[105]) illustrates how much we've distanced ourselves from our neurophysiological natures.

The final factor in assessing ideal bowel function is smell. When the digestive system is functioning optimally, the stool smell is relatively mild. If the odors are strong and overwhelmingly unpleasant, it's a sign that bacteria in the stool have been sitting and fermenting in the gut for too long—or that there's an imbalance in the gut bacteria. During the fermentation process, the stool produces gases that give off foul smells.

Though stool smell depends somewhat on nutrition and the bacterial balance in the body, it shouldn't be too intense if the bowels are working well.

IMMUNE FUNCTION AND THE NERVOUS SYSTEM

Besides its strong link to the digestive system, the nervous system is also closely connected with the immune system: the more time someone spends in a stressed out, sympathetic-dominant state, the weaker their immune system becomes.[106]

Along these lines, one of the telltale signs of a weak immune system is a frequent upper respiratory infection. Why?

The respiratory tract is a part of the body that interacts directly and frequently with pathogens in the environment. Since we breathe thousands of times a day, we're more susceptible to respiratory infections than any other type of infection.

If someone's immune system isn't functioning at full capacity, then they're especially vulnerable to upper respiratory infection. This is why frequent upper respiratory infections are often one of the first signs of a weak immune system.

Frequent upper respiratory infections are often indicative of imbalances in the nervous system, which can result from too much training, too little stimulation during training, and/or lack of physical or psychological resilience in handling stress.

LIFESTYLE-RELATED DISEASES AND THE NERVOUS SYSTEM

Just as upper respiratory infections are a sign of a weakened immune system and the lingering presence of too many stress hormones, chronic lifestyle-related diseases or issues like Type 2 diabetes[107] and high blood pressure[108] are often linked to excessive sympathetic nervous system activity. Simply put, these chronic conditions are usually a direct result of spending too much time in fight-or-flight mode.

For Diego, whose story kicked off this chapter, the combination of underlying health problems from years of taking excessive amounts of steroids for competitive bodybuilding, plus high stress levels, led to him developing chronic high blood pressure in his early thirties.

In the process of working with NeuFit, he learned new, more productive ways to cope with the stresses of modern life—and bring his body back into balance—by reeducating his brain and nervous system.

Four years after his initial training sessions, he continues to train regularly with the help of the Neubie. "Paying attention to things like heart rate variability and sleep has had a major impact on my health. It's also totally changed the way I work out," he said. "Now, I don't have to worry about pushing myself too hard. And I still don't need the beta-blockers to keep my blood pressure in a healthy range."

Diego's experience shows how valuable it can be to systematically monitor the health of the nervous system over the course of rehab and training. However, tracking the indicators of a well-functioning nervous system is just the first step. The next step is deciding what to do with this information.

Once someone has a clear picture of how their nervous system is functioning, what can they do to support recovery, adaptation, and optimal neurological health? So far, we've covered rehab and training approaches that improve neurological health. What about life outside the gym and the treatment room? How does lifestyle impact the health of the nervous system? This is the theme of Chapter 9.

9

THE NEUFIT METHOD
FOR LIFELONG
NEUROLOGICAL HEALTH

As a middle-distance runner on the track and field team at an Ivy League university, Molly was not only used to intense training—she actually enjoyed it. During the season and throughout the off-season, she prided herself on working out longer and harder than any of her teammates.

For years, Molly's dedication to track had paid off. But something shifted toward the end of her sophomore season: "I didn't change anything about the way I trained, and I hadn't had any serious injuries," she said. "But all of a sudden, I just had no energy at all."

By the end of the season, she was experiencing chronic bouts of fatigue. Her strength diminished, too, along with her speed. "By the time we got to the end of the season, I was dragging myself through workouts and meets. Pretty soon, I felt like I was dragging myself through life in general."

When she came home from college that summer, she forced herself to train, despite the fatigue. Every morning, she woke up feeling exhausted. Her bowel movements were irregular and often difficult to pass. Her heart rate variability was low. In short, there were multiple signs that something was off-balance in her nervous system.

Concerned about her health, she visited her family doctor, who performed a series of tests that revealed no underlying diseases or conditions. Though he encouraged her to rest, her doctor cleared her to continue training whenever she felt ready.

This was Molly's starting point when she came to NeuFit. Though her main goal was to get her speed and endurance back, we also wanted to focus on the bigger picture of her neurological health.

With this goal in mind, we not only designed a training program to improve her performance, but we also took a thorough inventory of her lifestyle. Why? As we explained to her, when it comes to performance—not to mention fitness and neurological health—our lifestyle choices play an essential role in supporting our training.

In other words, what we do in the other twenty-three hours of the day outside of training is just as important, if not more important, than what we do during training.

THE BODY BANK ACCOUNT

Over the course of working with Molly, we applied one of the concepts at the core of the NeuFit approach to rehab and training: the notion of the "body bank account." As with a traditional bank account, it's possible to make both deposits and withdrawals in the body bank account.

With the body bank account, the goal is clear: to build up the balance by making deposits—and compound the interest on those deposits with good habits and healthy lifestyle choices.

How does this idea work in practice? How do we categorize deposits or withdrawals in the body bank account? Things like proper breathing, good nutrition, and high-quality sleep represent deposits.

Withdrawals, meanwhile, can include things like watching television until two o'clock in the morning or drinking shots until closing time. Though there's nothing inherently wrong with these types of activities, it's important to recognize that they have a cost.

Since the body's recovery capacity is finite, using up this capacity for things like late nights or excessive alcohol consumption subtracts from the body's available balance for recovery from training.

Speaking of training, isn't it another deposit in the body bank account? It could be. But it depends on how someone trains. Many people, including Molly, assume that working out is a direct deposit when, in fact, it can be a withdrawal: breathing improperly during exercise, moving with poor form, and/or falling into a submaximal training pattern (i.e., doing too much or too little, as described in Chapter 6) are workout habits that ultimately detract from the body bank account.

This was exactly what was happening to Molly. In addition to working out past the point where she could exert maximum effort, she was sleeping poorly and disregarding her diet. In other words, her body bank account was seriously overdrawn—and her nervous system was showing all the signs.

Using the lifestyle strategies described in this chapter, we helped Molly restore the balance in her body bank account. Besides taking a neurology-first approach and emphasizing quality over quantity in her training, we expanded her focus to her health outside her workouts.

By paying attention to her breathing habits, general movement levels, nutrition choices, and sleep patterns, she not only improved her performance. She also made a significant positive impact on her neurological health.

THE POWER OF THE BREATH

Breathing is one of the most powerful influences on the body's ability to function at optimal capacity. Since the autonomic nervous system can regulate the breathing process without any conscious attention, most people assume they know how to breathe properly.

In reality, many people spend their days breathing in a way that slows them down, reduces brain function, causes them to store body fat, and negatively impacts their long-term health.

So how can people breathe better? There are two main factors to consider with breathing. The first is mechanics, which include using the nose and the diaphragm. The second is oxygen and carbon dioxide levels, which involve training the body to optimize its levels of carbon dioxide.

THE IMPORTANCE OF NOSE BREATHING

When it comes to improving neurological health, nose breathing is a good place to start. There are two main reasons why nose breathing is so important:

- Breathing through the nose plays a significant role in protecting the body from airborne pathogens.
- Breathing through the nose helps keep the body in, or closer to, a parasympathetic-dominant state.

Let's look at these reasons more closely. How does nose breathing protect the body from pathogens? Besides warming and moisturizing the air we breathe, the hairs and mucus membranes lining the nose and airways filter this air.

When pathogens get caught in the nose hairs and mucus membranes, they travel down the esophagus and into the stomach instead of going directly to the lungs. In the stomach, hydrochloric acid neutralizes these pathogens, stripping them of their potential to harm the body. In contrast, if we breathe through the mouth, airborne pathogens go straight to the lungs and increase the likelihood of respiratory infections.

Besides shielding the body from disease, nose breathing also has a direct impact on nervous system function. For example, studies led by Dr. John Douillard show that compared to mouth breathing, breathing through the nose during exercise increases heart rate variability and the proportion of alpha brain waves (which help the body stay calm, even during an exercise challenge).[109] Plus, Dr. Douillard found that participants in the study improved their endurance even though they were breathing less (I'll explain why in the sections below on carbon dioxide).

For now, it's important to understand why nose breathing has such a profound effect on the autonomic nervous system. One theory goes back to an association we make as babies. When babies are born, they're what's referred to as "obligate" nose breathers[110]—or at least "preferred" nose breathers.[111] Translation: at first, babies only inhale and exhale through the nose since their mouths are intended for taking in mothers' milk.[112]

However, the first time a baby has a stuffy nose or any trouble breathing through the nasal passages, they automatically start to panic—until they realize they can breathe through the mouth. Over time, the mouth becomes a kind of safety release valve that they learn to associate with panic or a sense of suffocation.

As a result, no matter where they are on the autonomic spectrum, any time someone breathes through the mouth, they tend to move closer to the fight-or-flight side of the nervous system. So if the goal is to avoid spending too much time in a stressed-out, sympathetic-dominant state, breathing through the nose is an essential health habit to practice at rest *and* during exercise.

Breathing and Carbon Dioxide

Besides breathing through the nose, one of the most important breath-related practices for nervous system health is the act of slowing down the breath and reducing breathing volume in order to balance carbon dioxide levels in the body. Why does carbon dioxide matter?

Most people believe it's best to get rid of all carbon dioxide because too much carbon dioxide can be poisonous. Along these lines, they generally breathe too much or too quickly, ending up with too little carbon dioxide in their systems.

However, carbon dioxide actually serves some very important functions in the body. There are several reasons it's an essential element in nervous system function as well as overall health:

- Carbon dioxide dilates the blood vessels, so it plays a key role in healthy blood flow to the brain and body.[113]
- Carbon dioxide is required for oxygen delivery to the muscles and organs. (In the absence of carbon dioxide, oxygen remains attached to the red blood cells and doesn't get distributed to the target areas of the body. Low oxygen levels in the body's tissues and organs can lead to a myriad of health issues.)[114]
- Carbon dioxide helps stabilize the nerves and calm neurological hypersensitivity. (This is why we tell people to breathe into a paper bag if they have a panic attack. The paper bag collects the exhaled carbon dioxide, allowing them to inhale it in a higher concentration in order to soothe the nerves.)[115]

Though it might come as a surprise, the brain actually monitors carbon dioxide levels in the blood, not oxygen.[116] Whenever our cells are generating energy, they give off carbon dioxide as a byproduct of the metabolic process. As carbon dioxide levels accumulate in the blood, they eventually reach a threshold where the brain triggers the desire to take a breath to release excess carbon dioxide.

MEASURING CARBON DIOXIDE LEVELS

Besides understanding the benefits of having healthy (generally, higher) carbon dioxide levels, we also want to understand how to measure them. There are two tools we recommend.

The first tool is simple: a breath-holding test. Originally developed by Soviet doctor K.P. Buteyko, who used breath retraining to ease symptoms in asthma patients, the test is called a "Control Pause" and goes like this:

- Sit in a relaxed position and breathe at your usual pace for at least five minutes.
- At the end of a normal exhale (breathing out as much as possible without forcing it), pinch your nostrils, start a timer, and hold your breath. Don't let any air enter the nose or mouth.
- Measure the time until you experience a palpable urge to inhale.

When the time is up, your next inhale should feel relaxed. If you feel the need to gasp for air, you held the breath too long.

According to Dr. Buteyko, a score of fewer than twenty seconds is a sign of suboptimal health. Between twenty and forty seconds indicates enough oxygen delivery to support average health. Forty seconds and above is the goal and a sign of excellent health.[117] The best time to attempt the Control Pause test is shortly after waking up in the morning. This way, you can get a glimpse of your "default" carbon dioxide levels without any influence from conscious breathing.

The second technique we use to assess carbon dioxide levels is more technologically sophisticated. It's called capnography, and it involves using a ventilation device to measure the amount of carbon dioxide at the peak of an exhalation.[118]

Given in partial pressure, average capnography values of carbon dioxide are between thirty-five and forty mmHG (millimeters of mercury). Below 35 mmHg is considered low and usually correlates with suboptimal health. Meanwhile, a reading above 40 mmHg is usually a sign of an elite level of training and excellent health and resilience.

DEVELOPING GOOD BREATHING HABITS

For the majority of people, training the body to handle higher levels of carbon dioxide is one of the keys to long-term neurological health. There are two ways to do this:

- Breathing exclusively through the nose and slowing down the breath rate during exercise (which is probably the most convenient method)
- Breathing drills outside of exercise that train the body to breathe less

The average person breathes fourteen to eighteen breaths per minute, or 20,000 to 26,000 breaths per day. However, when at rest, a healthier average is between six and twelve breaths per minute.

Maintaining optimal levels of carbon dioxide involves more than taking fewer breaths. What's even more important is the overall volume of air. At rest, the average breath is about 500 milliliters for a typical male adult and 400 milliliters for a typical female adult. Ideal breathing volume is about four to eight liters per minute (which leads to ten to twelve breaths per minute on average, though lower breath rates are even better).[119]

How can people improve their breathing habits and learn to breathe less? There are a variety of approaches rooted in different health, movement, and spiritual traditions. Though the details differ, all of these approaches share one thing in common: conscious awareness and intentional control of the breath.

In the sections that follow, I describe some of the breathing drills that have proven especially effective for NeuFit patients and clients, helping improve both their breathing mechanics and carbon dioxide levels.

Diaphragmatic Breathing

Using the diaphragm instead of the ribs and neck muscles to breathe initially requires more energy. This is why many people don't do it.

However, one advantage of diaphragmatic breathing is that it helps oxygen reach the lowest regions of the lungs, where there's more blood and a greater exchange of oxygen and carbon dioxide. In the long run, the added energy investment of using the diaphragm pays off, with far greater oxygen absorption, which translates into higher energy levels and better nervous system function.[120]

Another advantage of diaphragmatic breathing is its effect on the vagus nerve.[121] Since the vagus nerve passes through the diaphragm, breathing diaphragmatically mechanically stimulates the vagus nerve, increasing the activity of the parasympathetic nervous system.

When breathing from the diaphragm, the expansion and contraction of the abdomen moves the visceral organs. Since these organs, along with part of the diaphragm,[122] are innervated by the vagus nerve, their movement also increases vagus nerve activity.

Along these lines, combining diaphragm breathing with nose breathing is particularly effective in stimulating the vagus nerve.

HOW DIAPHRAGMATIC BREATHING WORKS

How do we know if we're breathing from the diaphragm? Since it doesn't have sensory nerves, we can't feel it. So we have to observe it by watching the movement of the abdomen.

As Figure 9-1 shows, the diaphragm contracts downward on an inhalation, pushing on the visceral organs and expanding the abdominal cavity in all three dimensions. On the exhale, the abdominal muscles contract, creating upward pressure that pushes the diaphragm back to its resting position, forcing air out of the lungs.

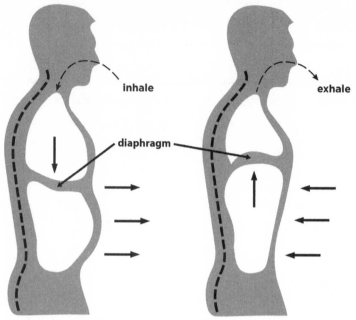

Figure 9-1: Diaphragmatic and abdominal activity while breathing.

To determine whether you're breathing from the diaphragm, try these steps:

- Sit or lie down.
- Place one hand on the chest, just above the sternum, and one hand over the belly button.
- Breathe in and out and observe which hand moves more.

If you're breathing through the diaphragm, there should be significantly more movement in the hand on the abdomen than the one on the chest.

This diaphragmatic breathing pattern should be the primary breathing pattern at rest and at low to moderate levels of activity, with the abdomen moving and the chest and neck remaining fairly still. When training hard, it's normal to add some amount of chest and neck breathing to allow for a greater volume of air.

TRAINING THE DIAPHRAGM FOR HIGHER PERFORMANCE

The strength or weakness of the diaphragm can have a major impact on performance. If the diaphragm gets fatigued, it starts to pull blood away from the other muscles, causing the entire body to fatigue. On the other hand, when the diaphragm grows stronger and more resilient, the body as a whole becomes more resilient and energy-efficient.[123]

Exercises that involve inhaling and exhaling against resistance are some of the best ways to strengthen the diaphragm muscles. At NeuFit, we like to introduce this concept manually, starting off with the simple practice of pinching the nostrils to reduce their size by about 50 percent and asking clients to breathe in. Inhaling through a smaller opening makes the diaphragm work harder. To experience a resisted exhale, we ask clients to breathe out through pursed lips. In order to push the air out through a smaller opening in their mouths, they usually have to activate the abdominal muscles.

Besides these manual techniques, there are three tools we recommend to practice inhaling and exhaling against resistance: the Relaxator (which works the muscles used during exhalation), the Breather (which creates resistance on the inhalation and exhalation but requires inhaling through the mouth) and the Training Mask (which also creates resistance on the inhalation and exhalation and has the added benefit of allowing you to breathe through the nose instead of the mouth). Appendix 2 has more information about all three of these tools.

IN THROUGH THE NOSE, OUT THROUGH THE MOUTH?

During or after an intense workout, trainers often suggest inhaling through the nose and exhaling through the mouth. However, there are some issues with breathing this way. When I ask coaches why they advise athletes to breathe in through the nose and out through the mouth, their answer is usually something like, "We've always done it that way." These are some of the most dangerous words in health, fitness, and medicine.

When exhaling through the mouth, people breathe out all of the carbon dioxide-rich air in the throat and upper chest. As a result, they end up blowing off more carbon dioxide (and reducing their levels of this important gas in the body).

When people exhale through the nose, they preserve more of that carbon dioxide-rich air in the upper throat and chest so they can take it in on the next inhale. Exhaling through the nose increases the amount of carbon dioxide in the body, which supports healthy blood flow and oxygen delivery, as well as balancing blood sugar and stabilizing the nervous system.

Air Hunger Drills to Optimize Carbon Dioxide Tolerance

As I mentioned earlier in this chapter, most people assume the brain monitors oxygen, though it actually monitors carbon dioxide levels far more closely. Again, it's when carbon dioxide levels reach a certain threshold that we experience the desire to breathe.

Air hunger drills—which involve slowing down the breath or holding the breath past the point of the urge to take the next breath—are designed to increase the amount of carbon dioxide in the body. By intentionally slowing down the breath and reducing the volume of air exchange, these drills train the brain and nervous system to stay relaxed even when the body is hungry for air—and teach the body to tolerate higher carbon dioxide levels.

People can practice air hunger drills naturally during physical activity. All they have to do is intentionally breathe through the nose and slow down the breath rate when the body reflexively wants to breathe through the mouth and speed up the breath rate.

I recommend starting off with air hunger drills during less strenuous activities, like walking. One way to do this is to synchronize the breathing with the walking stride, for example, by inhaling for four to eight steps and exhaling for eight to sixteen steps. After learning to control the breath while walking, people can progress to nose breathing and slowing the breath during more rigorous workouts.

Outside of training, practicing air hunger drills for as little as three minutes at a time can be valuable, particularly when done several times a day. Alternatively, bouts of ten to twenty minutes can also be effective if people practice consistently.

If people have trouble doing air hunger drills on their own, tools like the Relaxator (featured above in the section on diaphragmatic breathing and in Appendix 2) can help.

THE MASTER RESET

Together with the breathing practices outlined in this chapter, techniques like meditation and biofeedback are effective ways to strengthen the parasympathetic nervous system and build psychological resilience. With these goals in mind, NeuFit has developed a meditation-enhancing treatment known as the "Master Reset."

The Master Reset uses the Neubie to directly stimulate the vagus nerve. As explained in previous chapters, the vagus nerve controls the parasympathetic nervous system. More specifically, it governs crucial physiological functions like heart rate, breathing, and the communication between the digestive system and the brain. It also facilitates the body's relaxation response and affects the perceptions of threat that lead to pain (covered in Chapter 4).

During a Master Reset, patients lie down, and we place the Neubie's pads at specific locations on the body, including the base of the skull near the brain stem (where a series of cranial nerves, including the vagus nerve, exit the brain).

The other electrodes can go on the feet or hands (which are especially neurologically rich), or on the lower back (sending the current through the viscera and along the length of the spinal cord).

As the machine stimulates the nerves, we ask clients to breathe slowly and intentionally. For most people, just ten minutes of using this technique improves heart rate variability and activates the growth and regeneration processes of the parasympathetic nervous system.

It's certainly possible to do ten minutes of breathing practices without the Neubie and experience meaningful physiological and psychological benefits. At the same time, using the Neubie in treatments like the Master Reset can make it easier for patients to improve parasympathetic nervous system function and create a more significant neurological shift in a relatively short time.

Additional Breathing Exercises

In addition to the techniques I've outlined so far, there are two more breathing exercises we regularly recommend at NeuFit to improve neurological health: box breathing and doubling the exhale.

Box breathing involves inhaling for a count of four, holding the breath for four, exhaling for four, and holding for four over a period of several minutes or up to half an hour. Over time, the goal is to increase the count to eight or ten, with the length of each breath and hold remaining equal.

Doubling the exhale is an exercise that is as it sounds: breathing in for a certain count (like five to ten seconds) and then breathing out for twice as long (ten to twenty seconds). No matter how long the breaths, the aim is to make the exhalation twice as long as the inhalation. Why? Because the exhale is the phase of the breath that activates the parasympathetic nervous system. As I mentioned above, this exercise can also be combined with walking, using the steps to count the length of the breaths.

When people practice them consistently, both of these exercises help strengthen the parasympathetic nervous system and optimize carbon dioxide levels in the body.

BREATHING FOR DISEASE PREVENTION

Besides contributing to neurological health, good breathing habits can also play a role in preventing diseases like high blood pressure and cancer.

In numerous studies, high blood pressure patients who practiced focused breathing for twenty minutes a day saw reductions in blood pressure the same as or more significant than those who took beta-blockers or similar medications.[124]

Research also indicates that proper breathing may help counteract cancer, since reduced oxygen in the internal environment actually promotes the growth of tumors.[125]

KEEP ON MOVING

On top of good breathing habits, general, low-level physical activity outside the gym is another key to improving performance and sustaining neurological health.

In earlier chapters, we established how important consistent, nervous system-stimulating exercise is for long-term health and fitness. However, if optimal neurological health is the goal, an hour a day in the gym isn't enough. Besides working out regularly, it's important to move the body frequently throughout the rest of the day.

After a hard workout, being sedentary for most of the day can actually *undo* many of the benefits of exercise. And this doesn't just impact speed and strength—it can actually affect long-term health. A recent study of meta-data from more than one million people published in *The Lancet*, for example, showed that excessive sitting is linked with increased all-cause mortality.[126] (Interestingly, researchers in this study also identified high levels of television viewing time as a predictor of early death.)

Why is being sedentary so bad for our health? And how exactly does too much sitting affect the brain, nervous system, and the body as a whole?

THE CONSEQUENCES OF INACTIVITY

Leading a mostly sedentary life can cause a range of health problems, including:

- Blood sugar dysregulation, which can eventually lead to a series of health issues, including diabetes and cardiovascular disease[127]
- Muscle atrophy and loss of strength[128]
- Stagnation of blood and lymphatic flow (which blocks the removal of bodily waste products, triggering immune reactions that can cause serious inflammatory problems)[129]

Besides contributing to health problems like these, inactivity directly affects the brain and nervous system. If a person decides to sit on the couch all day, for example, their body quickly realizes it's producing more energy than it needs. The result? The brain sends signals to the body to downregulate energy production and metabolic function.

Why does this happen? Once again, it goes back to specificity of adaptation, a concept we covered in Parts 1 and 2 of this book. If someone spends most of their time sitting, the brain and nervous system respond and adapt accordingly. In the absence of movement or stimulation, the body automatically shifts into doing the minimum necessary for survival.

What are the actual neurological consequences of spending too much time in a chair? Over time, coordination and sensation become impaired, sensory or movement ability gets compromised, and the brain's overall functional capacity decreases.

How does someone know whether they need to incorporate more movement into their daily routine? It starts with doing a neurological system check, running the body through the indicators of nervous system health outlined in Chapter 8.

If factors like heart variability, sleep quality, digestion, and energy levels are pointing toward poor nervous system function—and it's clearly not a case of too much training—then there's a good chance that inactivity is part of the underlying problem.

INTEGRATING MOVEMENT INTO DAILY LIFE

As author and high-performance coach Brendan Burchard said, "A power plant doesn't *have* energy, it *generates* energy."[130] The same goes for the human body.

With this idea in mind, how can people use general movement to generate more energy—and improve their neurological health?

The following is a list of simple movement-generating techniques we recommend to NeuFit patients and clients, especially the ones who are sedentary most of the time outside of their treatment or training sessions:

- **Set an hourly alarm and take a five-minute walk every time it goes off.** Taking regular breaks like this is good for the mind as well as the body.
- **Practice micro-movements** throughout the day. Minor movements like kicking the foot, shifting the weight, or rotating back and forth in a swivel chair actually increase caloric demand and improve overall health.[131]
- **Switch positions.** Returning to the "use it or lose it" principle discussed in earlier chapters, regularly shifting bodily positions helps maintain range of motion and mobility, even from a seated position. For example, while sitting at a desk, regularly alternating the cross of the legs can make a difference. In a home working environment, going from a chair to sitting on the ground to lying on the stomach is helpful, too.
- **If possible, shift to a standing desk.** Standing demands more muscle engagement than sitting, especially in the leg muscles. Besides providing an opportunity for more micro-movements than sitting, standing can lead to better posture because it requires more intention (since there's no chair for the body to lean back on).
- **Find other ways to walk more.** Some people get treadmill desks. I enjoy taking phone calls or having meetings while walking outside. (There are additional health benefits to getting fresh air and natural sunlight, too.)

As people incorporate these general movement techniques into their daily routines, it's important to note how they affect the indicators of nervous system health. More often than not, people who spend the majority of their time being sedentary notice tangible improvements fairly quickly. If they don't see results, then it's usually a sign that they're already getting enough general activity—or that something else is off balance in the body.

THE POWER OF POSTURE

Along with integrating consistent general movement into daily life, practicing healthy posture is a simple but powerful way to maintain energy and boost neurological health.

Based on the principles of physiological psychology, if someone is sitting or standing erect with the head held high and the chest open, their energy level—and confidence—tends to be higher than that of a person who's slouching, rounding the shoulders, and collapsing the chest.[132]

Ultimately, a person's body position can have a profound effect on their mental and physical energy level. In other words, the simple act of shifting the posture can actually change the amount of energy in the body.

If you're hunched over reading this book, try standing up tall and puffing up your chest for one minute. Do you notice a difference in how you feel?

NUTRITION FOR NEUROLOGICAL HEALTH

While optimal nutrition varies based on individual requirements and goals, there are certain nutritional principles that apply across the board when it comes to supporting the nervous system, including:

- The need for adequate healthy fat
- The need to maintain relatively stable blood sugar
- The need for minerals and other micronutrients that support neurological health
- The need for proper hydration
- The need to integrate nutrition into a sustainable daily routine

In this section, we'll cover best practices around each of these nutritional principles and explore their implications for long-term neurological health.

THE THING ABOUT FAT

Consuming adequate fat is crucial for overall health, as well as the health of the brain and nervous system.

Though often vilified, fat is a good source of energy. Oxidizing one molecule of fatty acid yields over one hundred molecules of ATP (energy in the form used by the body's cells), while a glucose molecule yields just thirty-eight molecules of ATP.[133]

Without enough fat, the body's metabolic and hormonal systems can't function at full capacity. How does this affect the brain and nervous system? In terms of metabolic health, too little fat—or too many of the wrong fats—can lead to an overreliance on carbohydrates for energy and related problems with blood sugar dysregulation. Among other issues, blood sugar dysregulation can cause inflammation in all areas of the body, including the brain. Over time, inflammation in the brain can have a negative impact on cognitive processes and overall nervous system function.

Besides helping to balance the blood sugar and ease inflammation, fat is also a major building block of the hormones, including testosterone and growth hormone,[134] which are essential for repairing and rebuilding the body after exercise or injury. And cholesterol has some significant benefits, too: it can help neurological patients repair and remyelinate damaged nerves,[135] prolong the survival of ALS patients,[136] and reduce the risk of dementia.[137] Cholesterol also supports recovery from exercise and helps people maintain strength and muscle mass as they age.[138] This is why statin drugs, which lower cholesterol, can have negative effects on the integrity of muscle and connective tissue as well as hormones.[139]

On top of this, every cell membrane in the body is composed of fat, and the cells need fat to support their renewal. Over the course of a person's life, the cells are continuously regenerating: every few days, the body recycles its gut lining. Every thirty days, the body recycles skin cells. Every eight months or so, virtually all of the body's cells replenish themselves. Again, each one of these cells needs high-quality fat to form healthy membranes.

MISUNDERSTANDINGS ABOUT FAT

What types of fats does the body need to function optimally? How much fat should a person consume? Before covering these basics, let's clear up some common misconceptions about fat.

Since the 1950s, much of the popular thinking around fat has centered on the idea that dietary fat and cholesterol are unhealthy. The idea that eating more fat and cholesterol directly increases fat and cholesterol levels in the body dates back to a physiologist named Ancel Keys. Keys linked the high rates of obesity and heart disease among people in the U.S. to higher fat and cholesterol consumption.

However, there's a large body of more current research that debunks Keys's claims, demonstrating that fat and cholesterol in the diet and in the blood don't cause cardiovascular disease. What actually causes cardiovascular issues is damage to blood vessel walls due to high blood pressure and/or circulating inflammation.[140]

Along the same lines, Stanford University neurology and biology professor Robert Sapolsky argues that damaged or inflamed blood vessels are a better predictor of cardiovascular problems than the amount of fat circulating through the veins. As long as there are no damaged vessels for harmful substances to stick to, Sapolsky says, a person could eat a dozen eggs a day "and have no worries in the atherosclerosis realm."[141] (Though I tried this at an earlier point in my athletic career, I don't generally recommend eating so many eggs unless athletes need them to fuel extreme amounts of training.)

A more recent study by researchers at the University of Connecticut and Ohio State University also disproves the idea that eating high levels of saturated fat is connected to obesity and cardiovascular disease—and that higher amounts of dietary fat cause higher levels of fats in the blood.[142]

Participants in the study consumed different ratios of fat and carbohydrates for several weeks at a time. Ultimately, researchers found that participants with the lowest amount of fat and cholesterol in their blood were eating the highest amount of fat and the least amount of carbohydrates. Meanwhile, those with the highest levels of fat in the blood were eating the highest amount of carbohydrates and the least amount of fat.

In other words, what goes into the mouth doesn't go directly into the blood, and this includes fat.[143] Instead, everything we eat gets filtered through the digestive tract. For this reason, the most important thing to focus on in terms of nutrition is consuming the right raw materials—including the right fats—so the digestive system can distribute them in the most effective way.

WHAT ARE THE "RIGHT" FATS?

When it comes to overall health—especially neurological health—certain types of fats are helpful, while others can be harmful.

In general, the body's cells need both saturated and mono-unsaturated fats for regeneration and growth. Why are these fats helpful? Since they're chemically stable, they provide the raw materials the cells primarily use.

Healthy sources of saturated and mono-unsaturated fats include grass-fed beef, pasture-raised chickens and their eggs (eggs with orange-tinted yolks are better than those with pale yellow yolks), olive oil, and avocado.

Meanwhile, polyunsaturated fats—from sources like canola and soybean oil that are high in omega-6 fats—can wreak havoc on the brain, nervous system, and overall health. Since they're chemically unstable, these polyunsaturated fats cause inflammation, which can lead to things like heart disease and stroke.[144] (Though they're also polyunsaturated, omega-3 fats from sources like wild-caught salmon and other fish, flaxseed, and nuts do provide health benefits.)

Trans fats, contained in partially hydrogenated vegetable oils, margarine, and many processed foods, are also damaging.[145] When cell membranes absorb trans fats, it becomes harder for the cells themselves to take up glucose from the blood, which can cause metabolic problems. Trans fats also make it harder for the liver to get rid of toxins in the body. All of this increases inflammation, which interferes with brain function and diminishes overall health.

HOW MUCH FAT DOES THE BODY NEED?

As with all of the recommendations outlined in this chapter, there's some individual variability in terms of how much fat people need. Different people will respond differently to various types of fats, particularly saturated fats, which are difficult to digest for some. What's more, some people may have allergies or sensitivities that affect how they react to certain foods.[146]

In general, it's important to keep in mind that the body requires energy from healthy fat sources to support metabolic, hormonal, and cellular health, as well as control inflammation. How much energy? This depends on a person's size, activity levels, and overall goals.

When adding more fats or making any significant dietary changes, we need to monitor how the body responds by observing the indicators of nervous system health outlined in Chapter 8. This information can help people decide how much fat they need to live and perform at their peak.

And what about carbohydrates? To be clear, I'm not advocating "no-carb" diets. When it comes to energy supply, the main goal is to keep the blood sugar stable. From a neurological perspective, it's possible—and much more sustainable—to have a healthy diet that includes some carbohydrates. See the "General Carbohydrate Recommendations" callout box, where I outline my favorite framework for determining appropriate amounts of carbs.

GENERAL CARBOHYDRATE RECOMMENDATIONS

How many carbohydrates does a person need to maintain and promote neurological health? As with fats, the precise amount varies according to their size and activity levels. However, there are some basic guidelines that help determine how many carbohydrates people need.

In *The Primal Blueprint*,[147] author Mark Sisson introduces a concept called the carbohydrate curve, which outlines optimal levels of carbohydrate consumption based on a person's starting point and goals.

For those who want to burn fat (technically, oxidize fat) and lose weight quickly, zero to fifty grams of carbohydrates per day is the goal, but it's not sustainable. For slower, more sustainable weight loss, fifty to 100 grams per day is a healthy range.

People who want to maintain their weight should shoot for 100 to 150 grams daily. For every hour of activity, adding another fifty to 100 grams of carbs is a good rule of thumb, depending on the intensity of the activity.

According to Sisson, most people consume between 150 and 300 grams of carbohydrates per day—well beyond what the body and nervous system of a sedentary or moderately active person needs to function. Over time, consuming carbs at this rate can lead to steady weight gain, not to mention blood sugar dysregulation and other metabolic problems.

MEAL TIMING AND INTERMITTENT FASTING

As I wrote in Chapter 8, when we're able to keep the blood sugar stable, we can go for longer periods between meals, creating the opportunity to experiment with techniques like intermittent fasting.

Though it may not be appropriate for athletes with intense training regimens (especially those looking to gain mass) or for people having trouble keeping up with other stressors in their lives, intermittent fasting can be beneficial. Besides promoting cellular repair in the nervous system,[148] intermittent fasting has been shown to reduce inflammation[149] and lower the risk of diseases like Alzheimer's and Parkinson's,[150] cancer,[151] cardiovascular disease,[152] and diabetes.[153]

The most common intermittent fasting strategy is known as 16:8. With this approach, people consume all of their meals for the day over an eight-hour period and fast for sixteen hours. Typically, this involves eating dinner around seven or eight in the evening and waiting until eleven or noon the following day to eat again.

There are certainly other ways to approach intermittent fasting. For example, I generally eat a large breakfast, fast for eight or more hours during the day, and eat a large dinner relatively early in the evening so my stomach is empty by the time I go to sleep.

If people are looking to align their eating patterns even more closely with their circadian rhythms (which we'll cover later on in this chapter), it can be better to limit their eating window to breakfast and lunch only.

Skipping dinner frees up the organs from digesting food overnight, which leaves more energy for the restorative processes of sleep and tends to improve sleep quality. However, some people don't like this approach, since it means missing out on the social component of eating dinner.

Whichever intermittent fasting strategy people choose, I recommend using the sleep monitoring strategies from Chapter 8 to see for themselves how their eating patterns might be affecting their sleep quality.

MINERALS, SUPPLEMENTS, AND NERVOUS SYSTEM HEALTH

In terms of nutrition, minerals are vitally important for many aspects of health, including neurological signal transmission, hormonal optimization, metabolism, maintenance and repair of body tissues, and more.

Like vitamins, minerals are considered micronutrients—compounds that have nutritional value and are necessary for health but don't contain calories. Everyone needs micronutrients to sustain life. When treating an injury or training to improve performance, people need even more of them.

Ideally, people should be able to get all the nutrients they need from food. However, even if someone has a healthy diet with plenty of good fats and vegetables, they're still likely to be short on key nutrients. Due to soil depletion and the nature of modern agriculture,[154] it's virtually impossible for people to get all the nutrients they need for optimal neurological health from food alone.

Supplements can be an effective way to make up for nutrient deficiencies, though we don't want to rely on them too heavily (by definition, a supplement is "something that enhances something else when added to it."). Instead, the goal is to derive as much nutritional value as possible from food—and use supplements to literally supplement or enhance the diet.

Which supplements are important for supporting the brain and nervous system? Again, individual requirements vary based on health status, genetics, gut composition, and more. That said, quality multivitamin and multimineral supplements are beneficial for most people, as are prebiotic fibers.

Minerals like sodium, magnesium, potassium, and calcium are vital for the brain, muscles, heart, and bones.[155] While it's important to get enough of them, we also want to avoid overloading on these minerals. Vitamin D, a key component of central nervous system function,[156] is another supplement we frequently recommend at NeuFit. Though it's better for the body to get Vitamin D from sun exposure, it's not always possible to get enough of it, especially in northern latitudes. Adequate B vitamins are also very important for a healthy nervous system.[157]

Taking probiotics can be worthwhile, too, but their effectiveness depends on whether they can survive stomach acids, as well as the bacterial composition in the gut (more on this in Appendix 2). Many people can also benefit from newer, lesser-known supplements like CoQ10 and PQQ, which have neuroprotective effects and can help improve brain function.[158]

How do people decide which supplements they need? To determine their individual requirements—and avoid spending money on supplements without knowing whether they're actually helping—I recommend working with a functional or integrative medicine practitioner.

Generally, adding trace mineral drops to filtered water is an effective way to incorporate supplements into a nutritional routine (see Appendix 2 for my recommendations).

HYDRATION AND THE NERVOUS SYSTEM

Drinking plenty of high-quality filtered water isn't just important for general health. It's also a vital component of physical performance and cognitive function. According to a study published in the *Journal of Clinical Endocrinology and Metabolism*,[159] drinking 500 milliliters (16.9 ounces) of water increases a person's metabolic rate by 30 percent.

Though the effects of chronic or acute hydration are common knowledge, mild dehydration is a frequent problem that often flies under the radar.

Dehydration, even mild dehydration, limits energy production. If the body doesn't have enough water to take care of its basic survival functions, then there isn't enough left for higher-level cognitive tasks or elite athletic performance.

When I'm having trouble paying attention in a meeting, for example, it's often because I'm dehydrated. After drinking a large glass of water, I notice I can think clearly again within minutes.

On the other hand, there are risks associated with overhydration, which happens when the body takes in more fluids than the kidneys can remove. In other words, it's also possible to drink too much water.

The Ideal Amount of Water

How much water does a person actually need? Ultimately, the sense of thirst is our best guide. However, when we're going about our busy lives, it's easy to ignore our thirst, so it's helpful to have some basic guidelines.

A good hydration baseline is half to three-quarters of an ounce of water per pound of body weight. This translates to a minimum of sixty to ninety ounces per day for someone who weighs 120 pounds. For a person who weighs 200 pounds, 100 to 150 ounces a day is the minimum.

On hotter days, people need to drink more water because they're losing more water. When they work out, they also need to drink more. How much more? It depends on how much water they sweat out during exercise.

For example, a gallon of water weighs 8.3 pounds. If someone loses ten pounds of water during a workout (which can happen in a single hour when exercising in the heat[160]), then they need to drink more than a gallon to replenish that loss. When in doubt, urine color is a good indicator of hydration levels: clear to light yellow urine is a sign that someone is drinking enough water; dark yellow urine points to dehydration.

Why Drink Filtered Water?

Even in places with a healthy water supply, chlorine and fluoride are often added to water to prevent tooth decay and kill bacteria. Unfortunately, both of these substances can have negative health consequences. Excessive fluoride increases the potential for thyroid problems.[161] Chlorine has been linked to numerous health issues, such as an increased risk of cancer,[162] as well as problems with fetal development[163] and the immune system[164].

To remove these and other potentially damaging substances from water, I recommend a reverse osmosis filter. With its fine filtration system, reverse osmosis removes fluoride, whereas Brita pitchers or similar filters generally don't. However, since reverse osmosis also removes some of the minerals necessary for neurological health, it's best to add them back in. (See Appendix 2 for my mineral supplement recommendations, and also consider drinking untreated spring water, which is high in natural minerals.)

When it comes to filtered water, I encourage people to think of it like an insurance policy. Though it may or may not yield immediate benefits, it definitely helps mitigate risks in the long term.

BALANCING NUTRITION AND EXERCISE

What's the best way to balance nutrition with workouts to support the nervous system? When is the best time to eat before training? And what types of foods should people eat before and after training?

In general, if we're concerned about athletic performance, then it's important to have fuel in the tank before a training session. As I mentioned in previous chapters, if the brain senses that the body doesn't have enough energy to survive, it will limit output and inhibit performance. [165]

However, it's also important to avoid eating right before a workout. Why? The nervous system automatically directs most of its energy toward digestion after a meal, which takes away energy from the muscles for training.

How much time should people allow for digestion before a workout? If they're having a shake or a smoothie, thirty to sixty minutes are usually enough. With a more substantial meal, two to four hours are ideal. Generally, it's easy to tell if the body feels sluggish because it's still digesting food.

In terms of what to eat, it's better for the nervous system to consume more fat, protein, low-glycemic carbs, and vegetables before a workout and outside of exercise. The best time to eat moderate or high-glycemic carbs is within two hours after training. After a workout, high-glycemic carbs replenish energy stores; instead of building up as fat, they get channeled into the muscles and the liver.

Another factor to keep in mind with respect to nutrition and timing is that digestion is typically more effective earlier in the day.[166] This is why it's better to eat larger meals in the morning and toward midday, and lighten up on meals in the evening. Since digestive processes slow down at night, having a big meal before bed tends to interfere with sleep quality.

SLEEP PRACTICES FOR LONG-TERM NEUROLOGICAL HEALTH

In Chapter 8, we established the importance of sleep for long-term neurological health. To recap: sleep quality matters just as much, if not more than, sleep quantity. And a good goal for high-quality sleep is to spend at least 50 percent of sleep time in a combination of deep and REM sleep.

What's the best way to achieve high-quality sleep? There are two main components:

1. Training in a way that stimulates the nervous system and triggers neurological recovery processes, as outlined in Chapters 1 through 7.
2. Building healthy sleep habits.

When it comes to building healthy sleep habits, there are many things people can do, including:

- Aligning with circadian rhythms
- Limiting or eliminating blue light after dark
- Creating a sleep-friendly environment

ALIGNING WITH CIRCADIAN RHYTHMS

Sleep is generally better when it's in sync with circadian rhythms—the twenty-four-hour sleep-wake cycle directed by the brain. Since circadian rhythms primarily respond to light and darkness in the environment, most people benefit from aligning their sleep cycles with the light and dark cycles of the day.[167]

According to a study of night-shift workers led by Dr. Raffa-ello Furlan,[168] sleeping out of sync with circadian rhythms increases sympathetic nervous system activity and triggers the body's stress response.

Virtually all of the participants in Dr. Furlan's study reported high rates of blood sugar dysregulation, digestive problems, high blood pressure, poor immune system function, and reproductive issues—all of which can be traced back to imbalances in the autonomic nervous system. On top of this, other researchers have found that being at odds with circadian rhythms impairs the ability to learn.[169]

The bottom line is this: going to bed earlier, i.e., as close to sundown as possible, helps the vast majority of the population sleep better. Since this isn't possible for everyone, there are ways to limit light exposure after dark that can help people align more closely with their circadian rhythms, improve sleep quality, and boost long-term neurological health.

A CIRCADIAN RHYTHM SLEEP EXPERIMENT

Are you skeptical about the benefits of going to bed earlier? If so, I encourage you to try this experiment: for one week, turn off the lights and go to sleep within an hour after sunset. (To experience the full effect, I recommend finishing your last meal at least three hours before bed.)

As the week progresses, observe your body's response:

- How do you feel when you wake up? How does waking up feel as the days go by?

- How is your heart rate variability?

- How is your energy level throughout the day?

- Do you notice any changes in your appetite?

- How is your digestion?

- Do you notice changes in your ability to think clearly?

More often than not, the simple act of going to bed with the setting sun leads to positive changes in all of these areas, all of which affect—and are affected by—nervous system health.

LIMITING BLUE LIGHT EXPOSURE

Eliminating or limiting blue light exposure after dark is one of the most effective ways to align the body more closely with its circadian rhythms. What is blue light and why does it have such a significant impact on circadian rhythms and sleep?

Blue light is a big component of sunlight during daylight hours, when the sun is high and bright in the sky. Blue light increases alertness, reaction times, and mood; it also pauses the production of melatonin (the hormone that regulates sleep). Toward the end of the day, blue light fades, and the sun gives off infrared light, reactivating melatonin production and signaling the body that it's time to power down and prepare for sleep.[170]

Before the advent of electricity, the sun was the only source of blue light for human beings. Thanks to artificial light sources, especially fluorescent lights, most people in modern society take in heavy doses of blue light after dark, which disrupts their natural sleep patterns, contributes to sleep disorders, and can lead to other significant health issues like obesity, cardiovascular disease, depression, and even cancer.[171] Laptop and smartphone screens, which emit high levels of blue light, intensify the problem.

Given that any exposure to blue light after sunset limits sleep quality, the best thing people can do to improve sleep is turn off all screens after dark. Of course, this isn't doable (or desirable) for everyone in this day and age. However, there are tools like blue-light-blocking glasses, along with smartphone apps and computer software that modify screen colors to help reduce or eliminate blue light—and go a long way toward helping people sleep better.[172] (See Appendix 2 for my recommendations.)

ADDITIONAL SLEEP HYGIENE TIPS

Besides going to sleep earlier and limiting blue light exposure, consistent bedtimes and waking times are another key to improving sleep quality. When people constantly vary the time they go to bed or wake up, it increases the production of stress hormones in the body. In fact, its effects on the nervous system are similar to those of night-shift work when it comes to functions like digestion, heart rate variability, blood sugar, and cognitive function.

A person's sleep environment also plays an important role in sleep quality. For one thing, the room should be as dark and quiet as possible. Temperature is important, too, since there's a circadian component to body temperature just as there is for light and energy. In other words, when body temperatures vary significantly throughout the night, it can have negative effects on sleep similar to blue light.

According to research published in *Current Opinion in Physiology*, lower body temperatures during sleep can help minimize energy expenditure and support energy reallocation, which can contribute to better sleep, not to mention better health.[173]

CIRCADIAN RHYTHMS AND TRAINING TIMES

Given the profound effects of sleep on the nervous system, what's the best way to integrate training into a healthy circadian rhythm? Some of the best research on this topic dates back to the work of Soviet sports scientists from the 1970s. To help their athletes achieve peak performance, Soviet researchers came up with some groundbreaking ideas about balancing sleep and training times that still hold true.

When asked why Soviet weightlifters consistently outperformed their U.S. counterparts at the Olympics, a Soviet coach replied,[174] "The Americans...went to bed later, around midnight or 24:00. They also got up later, around nine or ten. And they skipped their morning gymnastics."

For the Soviets, outdoor morning warm-ups were mandatory. They organized the rest of their training routine according to circadian rhythms: after their morning warm-up, athletes typically worked out three to four hours after waking up, between eight and eleven o'clock in the morning. Evening training sessions took place between four and six o'clock.

Building on the Soviets' research, other sports scientists have found that it's also possible to train the body to work out at other times—right after getting up, for example, or at lunchtime. In these cases, the key is to do it consistently. This way, thanks to specificity of adaptation, the body adjusts its digestive and energetic processes to align with circadian rhythms.[175]

NEUROLOGICAL HEALTH GOES BEYOND TRAINING

When it comes to fitness, performance, and long-term neurological health, training is just one piece of the puzzle—albeit a vital piece.

How someone prepares for and supports their training is just as important as their training itself, as Molly's experience illustrates.

Over the course of her work with NeuFit, Molly (the middle distance runner whose story started this chapter) came to understand what a profound impact her lifestyle choices were having on her performance, not to mention her neurological health.

"As long as I wasn't breathing properly, eating well, or getting a good night's sleep," she said, "My body wasn't ready to train."

"Instead of eating pasta every night and being so focused on carbs, I started having protein, good fats, and veggies," she added. Instead of staying up until two in the morning on my iPad, I went to bed before ten o'clock, which wasn't easy at first. But pretty soon I started to notice some big changes. It got easier after that."

By the end of the summer, Molly got her energy back. Along the way, she increased her vertical jump by three inches and her squat by thirty pounds. She also gained five pounds of muscle and lost 2 percent body fat.

By giving her body the resources to make the most of her workouts, Molly made major improvements to her performance and went back to being a leader on the track team. By making lifestyle choices to support her training, she also laid the groundwork for a lifetime of neurological health.

CONCLUSION

The NeuFit Method harnesses the innate capacity of the brain and nervous system to generate immediate, profound, and sustainable results in rehab, fitness, and performance.

Since it controls every function in the body, the nervous system represents the clearest path to treating injury, chronic pain, and neurological injuries and diseases, as well as stimulating recovery post-surgery.

The same holds true for fitness and performance. Addressing the body's underlying neurological patterns helps people break through their self-imposed limitations and achieve new levels of strength, mobility, and resilience.

In contrast to conventional approaches to rehab and fitness, which tend to emphasize the body's hardware (i.e., the bones, tissues, and physical structure), NeuFit's focus on upgrading the body's software strategically stimulates the nervous system, creating a new set of neurological commands that accelerate recovery and boost performance.

DRAWING ON THE POWER OF ADAPTATION

Since the brain's number one priority is survival and protection, it often blocks the body's ability to heal and function in an optimal way. By drawing on the neurological capacity for adaptation and change, the NeuFit Method redirects the brain's energy and resources toward the long-term processes of rebuilding, replenishment, and growth.

No matter their starting point, every person's innate potential for positive adaptation represents an opportunity for faster healing (or at the very least some healing, if they haven't experienced any) and better performance.

In order to generate positive adaptation and long-term neuroplastic change, people need a strong physiological foundation. They also need the right kind of neurological stimulation. This is where the Neubie—NeuFit's patented, FDA-cleared electrical stimulation device—comes in.

Using the power of direct current, the Neubie closely approximates the natural frequencies of the nervous system, easing the body's stress response to electrical stimulation. In the process, it triggers the brain to connect with its inherent ability to regenerate and make beneficial adaptations, optimizing the process of neuromuscular re-education. (See Appendix 1 for more detailed information about the Neubie.)

THE NEUFIT METHOD FOR REHAB

When it comes to injury rehab (or any type of rehab, for that matter) the biggest obstacle to healing is often the body's *reaction* to the original trauma rather than the trauma itself.

In other words, in rehab and in life, it's not always about what happens to us but how we respond to it.

In the interest of survival, the brain works to protect traumatized areas of the body to prevent further injury. All of this protective tension and inhibition slows down the recovery process, limits movement, and actually increases the likelihood of re-injury. Even worse, these protective patterns often linger long after an injury has healed, leading to chronic pain and/or dysfunction.

Using muscle tests, manual muscle activation techniques, and body scans with the Neubie, NeuFit's approach to rehab pinpoints all of the areas where the brain's protective mechanisms are impairing function and blocking healing. Then we apply a combination of strategic movements and electrical stimulation from the Neubie to help the body to release its grip on the muscles, restore blood flow, and pave the way for fast, safe, and effective recovery.

THE NEUROLOGICAL APPROACH TO POST-SURGICAL RECOVERY

As is the case with injuries, the body's response to surgery often hinders the overall recovery process. Due to the trauma associated with surgery, the body's compensatory protective patterns after surgery tend to be more exaggerated than after injury.

By resetting the brain's trauma response after surgery, NeuFit treatments typically restore function much faster than conventional approaches to rehab. In the process, our approach also facilitates structural (hardware) healing. How? Upgrading the body's software—by removing the obstacles to recovery at the level of the brain and nervous system—frees up the body's resources to repair its physical hardware.

NEUFIT TREATMENT FOR CHRONIC PAIN

Regardless of its cause, pain is experienced in the brain rather than in the body. This is why working at the neurological level allows us to pinpoint the sources of chronic pain and treat them. Whether these sources of pain are physical or psychological, they show up as protective patterns in the body that we can identify and reset.

When combined with the electrical stimulation of the Neubie, the neurological approach to treating chronic pain goes to the roots to provide relief. In the absence of precise neurological stimulation, it's difficult to create such immediate, meaningful, or lasting results. The same is true for patients dealing with neurological injuries or diseases.

NEUROLOGICAL CONDITIONS AND THE NEUFIT METHOD

By shifting neurological inputs and facilitating healing at the functional level, we can reverse the effects of learned disuse and restore damaged nerve pathways in many patients with multiple sclerosis, spinal cord injuries, and traumatic brain injuries, as well as stroke and neuropathy patients.

By supplying the right kind of stimulus on the right neural pathways, we help patients with neurological conditions tap into their innate capacity for making neuroplastic changes. Sometimes, this is enough to help them recover sensation and mobility, as well as build strength, endurance, and resilience at the level of the nervous system.

MAKING THE TRANSITION FROM REHAB TO FITNESS

From a neurological perspective, transitioning from rehab to fitness training is more like walking up a gradual hill than leaping across a chasm. Instead of declaring rehab "complete," we recognize the overlap between effective rehab and effective training—and focus on evaluating each client's progress on a continuum. As their overall functional capacity increases, we increase the level of difficulty, even as we minimize the risk of injury (or re-injury).

THE NEUFIT METHOD FOR FITNESS TRAINING

NeuFit's approach to fitness training has two primary goals: 1) increasing neurological resilience, and 2) enhancing the quality of neurological stimulation.

Combining a tool like the Neubie with strategic, neurologically targeted movements makes it possible to safely yet significantly intensify the challenge during a workout—and achieve results more quickly than traditional approaches to training.

By enhancing the quality of neurological stimulation during training, we trigger the body's processes of optimal recovery, regeneration, and growth. In the process, we improve overall health. We also build resilience, teaching the body to remain in a healthy neurological state, even in the face of physical or psychological stress.

ELITE ATHLETIC PERFORMANCE AND THE NEUFIT METHOD

Regardless of their sport, all athletes need a certain level of basic movement proficiency, endurance, strength, and speed, in addition to their sport-specific skills, in order to compete at the highest levels. These traits are the building blocks of what we call the NeuFit performance pyramid.

Because of the brain's survival bias, it will often create limitations in all areas of the pyramid, which diminishes overall performance. When athletes invest in developing all areas of the pyramid at the neurological level, they not only create a strong foundation for elite performance, they also dramatically reduce their risk of injury and increase their chances of competing at the highest levels over the long term.

READING THE INDICATORS OF NERVOUS SYSTEM HEALTH

How does an athlete decide how hard to train? And how can people monitor the body's responses to training and rehab in general?

At NeuFit, we use a set of indicators of nervous system health to measure the body's response to rehab and training—and assess overall neurological health. Factors like heart rate variability, heart rate response to exercise, energy levels and libido, sleep quality, bowel function, immune function, body composition, appetite, and the presence (or absence) of chronic lifestyle-related diseases like high blood pressure and diabetes can give us valuable insights into nervous system function. This is why we use these indicators to shape our approach throughout the course of rehab and training.

INTEGRATED LIFESTYLE STRATEGIES FOR LONG-TERM NEUROLOGICAL HEALTH, FITNESS, AND HIGH PERFORMANCE

If the indicators of nervous system health point to neurological imbalances or poor nervous system function, it's important to reassess our approach to rehab and training. However, it's just as important—sometimes more important—to evaluate people's lifestyles outside the clinic or the gym.

Beyond training, there are four main lifestyle areas that have a major effect on neurological health: breathing, general movement, nutrition, and sleep. The choices people make in each of these areas can have a profound influence on their physiological and psychological state, the effectiveness of their training, the quality of their performance, and the long-term function of the nervous system.

THE NEUFIT METHOD FOR LIFE-LONG NEUROLOGICAL HEALTH

At every moment, the body's movements send signals to the nervous system. These signals either direct people toward good health and neurological growth—or chronic disease and diminished function.

By tapping into the natural capacity of the nervous system, the NeuFit Method gives people the tools to move toward greater vitality and peak performance. By rewriting self-defeating neurological programming, it opens up a range of new possibilities when it comes to rehab and fitness.

Combining the power of the Neubie with leading-edge approaches to recovery and training, NeuFit has enabled tens of thousands of people of all ages and abilities to unleash their natural physical potential—and set the stage for a lifetime of neurological health. Are you ready to discover what it can help you achieve?

To experience the NeuFit Method for yourself, or learn more

about the benefits of adding the Neubie to your practice, visit our website at www.neu.fit/book.

APPENDIX 1

THE NEUBIE

The Neubie (which stands for "**neu**ro-**bio**-electric stimulator) is the patented medical device at the core of the NeuFit Method for rehab and training.

The Neubie is FDA-cleared for the following uses:

- Maintaining or increasing range of motion
- Increasing local blood circulation
- Preventing atrophy
- Reducing spasms
- Preventing venous thrombosis after surgery
- Management or relief of chronic pain
- Management of post-surgical and post-traumatic acute pain
- Neuromuscular re-education

WHAT MAKES THE NEUBIE UNIQUE?

Its technical specifications are part of what makes the Neubie unique. By using direct current rather than alternating current, the Neubie maximizes the potential for neuromuscular re-education and improved neurophysiological function.

Beyond its effects on neuromuscular re-education and function, the Neubie's use of direct current can also promote tissue healing and repair. Whereas the alternating current in machines like TENS, NMES, Russian Stim, and Interferential creates electric fields that switch direction many times per second, direct current sustains an electric field in one direction for a longer period of time. This electric field can orient—and possibly increase—the activity of cells that repair and regenerate all types of tissues, including bone, muscle, and connective tissue.[176]

Besides using direct current, the Neubie's waveforms have been engineered to reduce resistance and irritation to the skin, along with the discomfort associated with electric charge accumulation (which often occurs with traditional direct current devices).

HOW THE NEUBIE FITS INTO THE NEUFIT METHOD

As interesting and unique as the Neubie's technology is, its benefits also come from integrating the device into the other components of the NeuFit Method, including assessments, exercises, and manual therapies.

Using the Neubie to map the body during an assessment, for example, offers unique insights into where the body is limiting itself due to perceived threats. In addition, it's possible to apply the Neubie while patients perform specific exercises, which enables clinicians to target movement patterns and increase the task specificity of treatment interventions.

Clinicians can also combine the Neubie with manual therapies, using their hands, various instruments, or what we call the "electric glove" to channel the device's current to strategic pressure points on the body. Many therapists and practitioners find that they're able to help tissues release faster and with less pressure by using the Neubie in addition to their manual techniques.

IS THE NEUBIE RECOMMENDED FOR EVERYONE?

The Neubie is not appropriate for patients who are pregnant or have pacemakers. In general, we encourage clinicians to exercise caution and use their professional judgment when using the Neubie with patients who have recent blood clots or cancerous tumors.

With blood clots and tumors, electric current itself isn't the primary risk. In these cases, the risks are associated with increasing blood flow—and possibly increasing metabolic activity—in the areas where the Neubie is applied.

WHAT PRACTITIONERS SAY ABOUT THE NEUBIE

Based on our own data and internal surveys of NeuFit providers, over 90 percent of patients experience tangible, positive results during their first treatment with the Neubie. For clinicians and practitioners, the ability to add value and serve patients at the highest level is the biggest motivating factor for incorporating the Neubie into their treatment protocols.

Many clinicians also see significant improvements in their business, which they typically attribute to their capacity to differentiate themselves and stand out within their communities.

In the meantime, we're constantly working to improve the Neubie, adding new features and new methods of application. To learn more about the device and about our latest innovations, visit the NeuFit website at www.neu.fit.

APPENDIX 2

RECOMMENDED TOOLS TO SUPPLEMENT NEUROLOGICAL HEALTH

In this section, I describe some of the additional tools and technologies we recommend and/or use at NeuFit. If you're interested in trying out any of these tools, you can find more information, links, and some discount codes at www.neu.fit/book.

RELAXATOR

Though people can effectively practice diaphragmatic breathing and air hunger drills on their own, these drills are potentially easier with the help of a device called the Relaxator. The Relaxator resembles a pacifier, and it's a small, convenient breathing retraining tool that people place in their mouths.

Equipped with an adjustable hole that slows down the exhale, the Relaxator is an easy way to train the body to slow the breath, reduce overall breathing volume, and build up higher levels of carbon dioxide in the body, which can have significant beneficial effects on health and performance. Like any training that involves reduced breathing, working with the Relaxator also builds resilience by helping people learn to stay calm—even when the brain has impulses to panic.

THE BREATHER

The Breather is an excellent tool for strengthening the respiratory muscles. It looks like a thick straw with a ball on the end. Though I don't like that it requires breathing in through the mouth, it does create resistance on the inhalation and exhalation muscles, so I still recommend it as a respiratory training device.

Using the Breather for ten to twenty breaths a day—especially if you breathe through the nose for the remainder of the day—is generally worth it. That said, it's best to use the Breather in an area with good air quality, e.g. outdoors in nature or in an indoor area with good air filtration. Avoid using it in the same room as someone with a respiratory illness.

TRAINING MASK

Like the Breather, the Training Mask is a tool that trains the respiratory muscles through resistance. It's an actual mask that covers the face, and it has valves that increase or decrease the resistance to inhalation and exhalation. My favorite thing about the Training Mask is that it allows breathing through the nose. Though you can use it for stand-alone breath training, I also like that you can wear it during activity.

OURA RING

The Oura Ring is a sleep and activity monitor that combines convenience with quality data. It has the form of a regular ring. (Besides using it as a tracking device, I wear mine as my wedding ring.) In addition to tracking sleep quality (in the form of time spent in light, deep, and REM sleep), it provides heart rate and heart rate variability measurements, breathing rate, and body temperature.

Though it tracks steps, too, the Oura Ring only counts them if the hands are moving while you're walking. (That is, if you're pushing a shopping cart or stroller, carrying a bag or a child, or doing anything that requires you to hold your hands steady while you walk, it won't count your steps—or at least it won't count them accurately.) Ultimately, I find its biggest value in sleep tracking.

BIOSTRAP

The BioStrap is a biometric tracking system similar to the Oura Ring. However, it has more features and a larger (but still convenient) format. Its wrist strap provides the same measurements as the Oura Ring during sleep, except for REM sleep. (There are some issues with the accuracy of REM tracking with wrist- or hand-based devices, though this functionality is improving and will likely be added by the time you read this book.)

The Biostrap also measures blood oxygen saturation and arterial elasticity (an important indicator of blood vessel health). It tracks movement, too, and it's especially accurate with step counting/activity tracking if you use the optional pod that fits on a shoe or around the ankle. One of its most powerful features: the Biostrap pairs with a forearm or chest strap that provides precise heart rate measurements during exercise, and it's sensitive enough to detect heart rates of 200 and above.

Overall, the Biostrap is probably the most accurate wearable biometric device on the market today. Readers of *The NeuFit Method* can get a discount on Biostrap products at www.bio-strap.com by entering the promo code NEUFIT at checkout.

TRACE MINERAL DROPS

If you drink reverse osmosis water (one of the nutrition strategies I discussed in Chapter 9), I recommend adding mineral drops to water to remineralize it. Why? In addition to filtering out many of the substances we don't want, reverse osmosis filters also remove many valuable minerals from drinking water. To replace these minerals, I like the ConcenTrace line of products by Trace Minerals, which are available online and at many grocery stores.

FOOD SENSITIVITY TESTS

Time and again, I've seen colleagues, clients, and patients relieve digestive problems, clear brain fog, increase energy, get rid of headaches and skin rashes, and/or improve sleep just by eliminating foods that were causing negative reactions.

How do you test for food sensitivities? One way is to follow an elimination diet, which involves removing certain foods from your diet for a period of time—generally between two and four weeks—and then adding them back in to see how they affect you. Typically, an elimination diet involves removing common allergens like wheat and gluten, cow's milk, eggs, peanuts, tree nuts, shellfish, and citrus fruits.

Blood tests are another way to identify foods that may not agree with you. If you work with a functional or integrative medicine practitioner, they can usually recommend one. There's also an excellent at-home option from a company called EverlyWell. Their tests involve a finger prick to provide a small blood sample, and they measure the body's immune response to ninety-six different foods.

If you happen to discover a food sensitivity, keep in mind that it may be possible to improve your digestive capacity and reincorporate that food in your diet later on. In the short term, however, removing any offending foods can free up a large amount of the body's energy. This is why exploring food sensitivities can be worthwhile if you're suffering from any unexplained health problems or energy deficits.

VIOME

Similar to food sensitivity tests, the Viome provides insights on how different foods affect your health. Unlike the Everlywell test, the Viome uses fecal samples rather than blood. With their at-home kit, you provide a small fecal sample and send it off for analysis.

The Viome test evaluates gut bacteria and the presence of other compounds like viruses and undigested food. It also provides information about digestive efficiency, inflammation levels in the gut, and even mitochondrial health. Based on the bacterial composition of your gut, the test recommends foods to eat and foods to avoid to improve your digestive health.

I like this test because of the growing evidence of how gut bacteria affects many aspects of health, including digestive function, brain function, mood and behavior, immune function and inflammation, stress levels, and metabolic health.[177]

If you'd like to take the Viome test, check out www.neu.fit/book for links and current discount codes.

FIVE FINGER SHOES AND OTHER MINIMALIST FOOTWEAR

Though we obviously need them for movement, the feet are also vitally important for neurological communication throughout the body. Wearing shoes with thick soles reduces the neurological input that we receive via the feet through walking. Over time, this reduced input can impair the brain and nervous system's ability to process input from the feet—and adversely affect balance.

This is why I strongly recommend "minimalist" footwear. To qualify as minimalist, shoes need to have a thin, flat sole (to qualify as thin, the sole should be flexible enough to allow you to bend the shoe or roll it up in your hand) and a toe box wide enough for the first and fifth toes to spread out in a healthy line with no compression.

My favorite minimalist footwear: the Five-Finger shoes from Vibram, which have a place for each toe and look like gloves for the feet. (I've been wearing these shoes virtually every day for ten years, and I swear by them.) If you don't like the look of Five-Finger shoes, there are a number of other excellent options, including Xero Shoes and Vivobarefoot, which I also wear.

BLUE LIGHT-BLOCKING PRODUCTS

As discussed in Chapter 9, exposure to blue light after dark can harm sleep quality by impairing melatonin production. Since it's not always possible to avoid screens and other sources of blue light after dark, I recommend two products to mitigate the effects of blue light on sleep and circadian rhythms.

The first is blue-light-blocking glasses, which have red or orange-tinted lenses. There are some inexpensive options available online that work well. I also like the TrueDark line of glasses. Visit www.neu.fit/book for current discount codes on TrueDark products.

In addition to glasses, I recommend software programs that reduce blue light on computers and tablets. Two that I particularly like are F.lux and Iris. Many smartphones, tablets, and computers also offer settings to reduce blue light.

ACKNOWLEDGMENTS

Briana, Gwenny, and Gemma, being with you brings so much depth and joy to my life and challenges me in the best ways possible. Queen Bri, thank you for helping me elevate my game in so many ways. Your influence is infused throughout the pages of this book, in our team and culture at NeuFit, and of course in all our marketing. I'm so grateful to you for supporting me through all the ups and downs on the journey of growing NeuFit and writing this book. Because of you, I'm a stronger person in so many ways.

Dad ("Boomer"), thank you for modeling generosity and professional excellence while still being an excellent father. Mom ("Mooti"), thank you for constantly encouraging me to be open to new ideas and go after my dreams, no matter how unattainable or crazy they seemed—and doing the same in your own life. Greta, your passionate pursuit of your music career has inspired me more than you know.

This book is rooted in the support of my family, and it's also a result of all the amazing learning opportunities I've had over the past fifteen years. I'm grateful to the mentors and teachers, patients and clients, and colleagues and friends I've had the opportunity to meet and interact with over the years. You've all made a contribution to this book.

There are a few mentors I'd especially like to acknowledge. Jaimen McMillan, founder of Spacial Dynamics, who taught me so much about movement and pedagogy, about how to be an effective leader and educator, and how to lead by example. Dr. John Pietila, my first neurology teacher, showed me what's possible when we apply neurology to rehabilitation and fitness. Dr. Eric Cobb, the founder of Z-Health, helped me see the breadth and depth of the effects we can have when working neurologically.

To my earliest colleagues in the "laboratory," Pricey, Kyle, and Rip (our honorary team member), I learned so much treating and training with you down in the dungeon.

To every person on Team NeuFit, thank you for all your incredible work. You've helped us grow from a 150-square-foot room to an international movement. I'm grateful, humbled, and thrilled by the impact that we're making. Special thanks to Ami, Kara, Ramona, Clay, Laura, Ruby, Leigh, and Earnie for keeping everything on track in the Neubie world so I could confidently step away to write this book.

To the entire community of NeuFit practitioners, thank you for putting your trust in our team and in me. It's an incredible honor to be able to work with you, and I can't wait to see what we continue to accomplish together.

To everyone who gave me permission to include their name

and/or story in this book, thank you. Working with you has made for some of the most humbling, gratifying, energizing, and rewarding experiences of my life. Brad Rowe, Trent Dilfer, Brent Burns, Dr. Terry Wahls, Dave Asprey, Anthony Rendon, Jason Waz, Whitney Jones, Dr. Ernie Bagnulo, Michele Harris, and Angie and Joe McGilvrey, I deeply appreciate you sharing your experiences and speaking up on behalf of our work at NeuFit. Ross, Amy J., Amy C., Ginger, Wendy, Tony, Talaya, Dawn, and Melinda, I'm also grateful to you for allowing me to share your remarkable stories.

Finally, Layne, thank you for your wonderful work on this book. You not only helped me clarify my ideas and weave in stories in a way that makes me feel truly proud of the finished product, you also helped me condense a 120,000-word behemoth into a book that I hope will be as accessible as it is inspiring for our readers.

ABOUT THE AUTHOR

GARRETT SALPETER combined training in neuroscience and engineering to start NeuFit, a company at the nexus of neurology and fitness, dedicated to treating athletes and patients in the realization of fitness goals, effective rehabilitation, and improved overall health. He is the host of *The NeuFit Undercurrent*, a podcast for patients and practitioners interested in learning more about neurology's role in recovery and performance. Garrett and his team have worked with thousands of patients recovering from neurological impairments, chronic pain, and sports injuries, including professional athletes, sports teams, and universities. He lives in Austin, Texas, with his wife and their two daughters.

REFERENCES

INTRODUCTION

1   The Neubie is FDA-cleared for the following uses: maintaining or increasing range of motion, increasing local blood circulation, neuromuscular re-education, preventing atrophy, reducing spasms, preventing venous thrombosis after surgery, management or relief of chronic pain, and management of post-surgical and post-traumatic acute pain. Since it uses the maximum power allowed by law in the United States, it also requires a prescription from a physician or the supervision of a licensed practitioner.

CHAPTER 1

2   Tor Nørretranders, *The User Illusion: Cutting Consciousness down to Size,* trans. Jonathan Sydenham (New York: Penguin Books, 1999).

3   Ingrid H. Sarelius et al., "Extracellular Matrix Fibronectin Initiates Endothelium-Dependent Arteriolar Dilatation via the Heparin-Binding, Matricryptic RWRPK Sequence of the First Type III Repeat of Fibrillar Fibronectin," *The Journal of Physiology* 594, no. 3 (January 15, 2016): 687–97, https://doi.org/10.1113/jp271478; Denise C. Hocking et al., "Extracellular Matrix Fibronectin Mechanically Couples Skeletal Muscle Contraction with Local Vasodilation," *Circulation Research* 102, no. 3 (February 15, 2008): 372–9, https://doi.org/10.1161/circresaha.107.158501; Daniel Goleman and Tara Bennett-Goleman, "Relieving Stress: Mind Over Muscle," *The New York Times*, September 28, 1986, https://www.nytimes.com/1986/09/28/magazine/relieving-stress-mind-over-muscle.html.

4   Eberhard Fuchs and Gabriele Flügge, "Adult Neuroplasticity: More Than 40 Years of Research," *Neural Plasticity* 2014 (2014): 1–10, https://doi.org/10/1155/2014/541870; Joyce Shaffer, "Neuroplasticity and Clinical Practice: Building Brain Power for Health," *Frontiers in Psychology* 7 (July 26, 2016), https://doi.org/10.3389/fpsyg.2016.01118; Patrice Voss et al., "Dynamic Brains and the Changing Rules of Neuroplasticity: Implications for Learning and Recovery," *Frontiers in Psychology* 8 (October 4, 2017), https://doi.org/10.3389/fpsyg.2017.01657.

5   Catherine E. Lang, Keith R. Lohse, and Rebecca L. Birkenmeier, "Dose and Timing in Neurorehabilitation," *Current Opinion in Neurology* 28, no. 6 (December 2015): 549–55, https://doi.org/10.1097/wco.0000000000000256; Laura Adomaitis Vearrier et al., "An Intensive Massed Practice Approach to Retraining Balance Post-Stroke," *Gait & Posture* 22, no. 2 (October 2005): 154–63, https://doi.org/10.1016/j.gaitpost.2004.09.001; Catherine E. Lang et al., "Observation of Amounts of Movement Practice Provided During Stroke Rehabilitation," *Archives of Physical Medicine Rehabilitation* 90, no. 10 (October 2009): 1692–8, https://doi.org/10.1016/j.apmr.2009.04.005.

6   Yihong Chen et al., "Physiological Electric Field Works via the VEGF Receptor to Stimulate Neovessel Formation of Vascular Endothelial Cells in a 3D Environment," *Biology Open* 7, no. 9 (September 15, 2018), https://doi.org/10.1242/bio.035204; Wei-Wen Hu et al., "The Effects of Substrate-mediated Electrical Stimulation on the Promotion of Osteogenic Differentiation and Its Optimization," *Journal of Biomedical Materials Research Part B Applied Biomaterials* 107, no. 5 (October 14, 2018): 1607–19, https://doi.org/10.1002/jbm.b.34253; Mahmoud Rouabhia et al., "Electrical Stimulation Promotes Wound Healing by Enhancing Dermal Fibroblast Activity and Promoting Myofibroblast Transdifferentiation," *PLoS One* 8, no. 8 (August 19, 2013), https://doi.org/10.1371/journal.pone.0071660; R. B. Borgens, J. W. Vanable, and L. F. Jaffe, "Bioelectricity and Regeneration. I. Initiation of Frog Limb Regeneration by Minute Currents," *Journal of Experimental Zoology* 200, no. 3 (June 1977): 403–16, https://doi.org/10.1002/jez.1402000310; Liudmila P. Leppik et al., "Effects of Electrical Stimulation on Rat Limb Regeneration, a New Look at an Old Model," *Scientific Reports* 5, no. 1 (December 17, 2015), https://doi.org/10.1038/srep18353; Colin D. McCaig et al., "Controlling Cell Behavior Electrically: Current Views and Future Potential," *Physiological Reviews* 85, no. 3 (July 2005): 943–78, https://doi.org/10.1152/physrev.00020.2004; Charles-Francois V. Latchoumane et al. "Chronic Electrical Stimulation Promotes the Excitability and Plasticity of ESC-Derived Neurons following Glutamate-induced Inhibition In Vitro," *Scientific Reports* 8, no. 1 (July 19, 2018), https://doi.org/10.1038/s41598-018-29069-3; Felix P. Aplin et al., "Ionic Direct Current Modulation for Combined Inhibition/Excitation of the Vestibular System," *IEEE Transactions on Biomedical Engineering* 66, no. 3 (March 2019): 775–83, https://doi.org/10.1109/tbme.2018.2856698.

CHAPTER 2

7   Stephanie M. Trigsted et al. "Greater Fear of Reinjury Is Related to Stiffened Jump-Landing Biomechanics and Muscle Activation in Women after ACL Reconstruction," *Knee Surgery, Sports Traumatology, Arthroscopy* 26, no. 12 (April 26, 2018): 3682–89, https://doi.org/10.1007/s00167-018-4950-2; Johan W. S. Vlaeyen et al., "The Role of Fear of Movement/(Re)Injury in Pain Disability," *Journal of Occupational Rehabilitation* 5, no. 4 (December 1995):235–52, https://doi.org/10.1007/bf02109988; Anna Trulsson et al., "Altered Movement Patterns and Muscular Activity during Single and Double Leg Squats in Individuals with Anterior Cruciate Ligament Injury," *BMC Musculoskeletal Disorders* 16, no. 1 (February 13, 2015), https://doi.org/10.1186/s12891-015-0472-y; Maaike Leeuw et al., "The Fear-Avoidance Model of Musculoskeletal Pain: Current State of Scientific Evidence," *Journal of Behavioral Medicine* 30, no. 1 (December 20, 2006): 77–94, https://doi.org/10.1007/s10865-006-9085-0; Johan W. S. Vlaeyen and Steven J. Linton, "Fear-Avoidance and Its Consequences in Chronic Musculoskeletal Pain: A State of the Art," *Pain* 85, no. 3 (April 2000):317–32, https://doi.org/10.1016/s0304-3959(99)00242-0.

8   Gabe Mirkin, "Why Ice Delays Recovery," DrMirkin.com, last modified September 16, 2015, https://www.drmirkin.com/fitness/why-ice-delays-recovery.html.

9   Julia M. Giger et al., "Rapid Muscle Atrophy Response to Unloading: Pretranslational Processes Involving MHC and Actin," *Journal of Applied Physiology* 107, no. 4 (October 2009): 1204–12, https://doi.org/10.1152/japplphysiol.00344.2009.

10 Markku Järvinen, "Healing of a Crush Injury in Rat Striated Muscle," *Acta Pathologica Microbiologica Scandinavica* Section A Pathology 83A, no. 3 (August 15, 2009): 269–82, https://doi.org/10.1111/j.1699-0463.1975.tb01874.x; Stefano Ciciliot and Stefano Schiaffino, "Regeneration of Mammalian Skeletal Muscle: Basic Mechanisms and Clinical Implications," *Current Pharmaceutical Design* 16, no. 8 (March 1, 2010): 906–14, https://doi.org/10.2174/138161210790883453; Tero A. H. Järvinen et al., "Muscle Strain Injuries," *Current Opinion in Rheumatology* 12, no. 2 (March 2000: 155–61,. https://doi.org/10.1097/00002281-200003000-00010; Tero A. H. Järvinen et al., "Muscle Injuries: Optimising Recovery," *Best Practice & Research Clinical Rheumatology* 21, no. 2 (April 2007): 317–31, https://doi.org/10.1016/j.berh.2006.12.004.

CHAPTER 3

11 David Andrew Rice and Peter John McNair, "Quadriceps Arthrogenic Muscle Inhibition: Neural Mechanisms and Treatment Perspectives," *Seminars in Arthritis and Rheumatism* 40, no. 3 (December 2010): 250–66, https://doi.org/10.1016/j.semarthrit.2009.10.001.

12 Julia M. Giger et al., "Rapid Muscle Atrophy Response to Unloading: Pretranslational Processes Involving MHC and Actin," *Journal of Applied Physiology* 107, no. 4 (October 2009): 1204–12, https://doi.org/10.1152/japplphysiol.00344.2009.

13 Atko Viru, "Post-Exercise Recovery Period," in *Adaptation in Sports Training* (New York: CRC Press, 1995)

14 Christopher V. Nagelli and Timothy E. Hewett, "Should Return to Sport be Delayed Until 2 Years After Anterior Cruciate Ligament Reconstruction? Biological and Functional Considerations," *Sports Medicine* 47, no. 2 (July 11, 2016): 221–32, https://doi.org/10.1007/s40279-016-0584-z; Stefano Zaffagnini et al., "Electron Microscopy of the Remodelling Process in Hamstring Tendon Used as ACL Graft," *Knee Surgery, Sports Traumatology, Arthroscopy* 18, no. 8 (September 29, 2009): 1052–8,. https://doi.org/10.1007/s00167-009-0925-7; S. Zaffagnini et al., "Neoligamentization Process of BTPB Used for ACL Graft: Histological Evaluation from 6 Months to 10 Years," *The Knee* 14, no. 2 (March 2007): 87–93, https://doi.org/10.1016/j.knee.2006.11.006.

CHAPTER 4

15 Though rare, CRPS is a debilitating disease that causes symptoms like acute pain spasms and extreme sensitivity to temperature, as well as significant reductions in movement.

16 Ronald Melzack, "Phantom Limbs and the Concept of a Neuromatrix," *Trends in Neurosciences* 13, no. 3 (March 1990): 88–92, https://doi.org/10.1016/0166-2236(90)90179-e; Asma Hayati Ahmad and Che Badariah Abdul Aziz, "The Brain in Pain," *Malaysian Journal of Medical Sciences* 21, Special Issue (December 2014): 46–54, https://pubmed.ncbi.nlm.nih.gov/25941463; Patrick D. Wall, "On the Relation of Injury to Pain the John J. Bonica Lecture," *Pain* 6, no. 3 (June 1979): 253–64, https://doi.org/10.1016/0304-3959(79)90047-2.

17 Katja Wiech, Markus Ploner, and Irene Tracey, "Neurocognitive Aspects of Pain Perception," *Trends in Cognitive Sciences* 12, no. 8 (August 2008): 306–13, https://doi.org/10.1016/j.tics.2008.05.005; M. N. Baliki, P. Y. Geha, and A. V. Apkarian, "Parsing Pain Perception Between Nociceptive Representation and Magnitude Estimation," *Journal of Neurophysiology* 101, no. 2 (February 2009): 875–87, https://doi.org/10.1152/jn.91100.2008.

18 Asma Hayati Ahmad and Che Badariah Abdul Aziz, "The Brain in Pain," *Malaysian Journal of Medical Sciences* 21, Special Issue (December 2014): 46–54, https://www.ncbi.nlm.nih.gov/pmc/articles/PMC4405805; Irene Tracey and Patrick W. Mantyh, "The Cerebral Signature for Pain Perception and Its Modulation," *Neuron* 55, no. 3 (August 2007): 377–91, https://doi.org/10.1016/j.neuron.2007.07.012; J. Talbot Get al., "Multiple Representations of Pain in Human Cerebral Cortex," *Science* 251, no. 4999 (March 15, 1991): 1355–8, https://doi.org/10.1126/science.2003220.

19 Beth D. Darnall, Daniel B. Carr, and Michael E. Schatman, "Pain Psychology and the Biopsychosocial Model of Pain Treatment: Ethical Imperatives and Social Responsibility," *Pain Medicine* 18, no. 8 (August 2017): 1413–5, https://doi.org/10.1093/pm/pnw166; Additional credit goes to Dr. Eric Cobb of Z-Health Performance Solutions for popularizing the metaphor of the threat bucket.

20 Haiou Yang, et al., "Low Back Pain Prevalence and Related Workplace Psychosocial Risk Factors: A Study Using Data From the 2010 National Health Interview Survey." *Journal of Manipulative and Physiological Therapeutics* 39, no. 7 (September 2016): 459–72, https://doi.org/10.1016/j.jmpt.2016.07.004; E. S. Nahit et al., "Effects of Psychosocial and Individual Psychological Factors on the Onset of Musculoskeletal Pain: Common and Site-Specific Effects," *Annals of the Rheumatic Diseases* 62, no. 8 (August 1, 2003): 755–60, https://doi.org/10.1136/ard.62.8.755.

21 Steven James Linton, "Occupational Psychological Factors Increase the Risk for Back Pain: A Systematic Review," *Journal of Occupational Rehabilitation* 11, no. 1 (March 2001): 53–66, https://doi.org/10.1023/a:1016656225318.

CHAPTER 5

22 Terry Wahls, *The Wahls Protocol: A Radical New Way to Treat All Chronic Autoimmune Conditions Using Paleo Principles* (New York: Avery, 2014).

23 Valentina Tomassini et al., "Neuroplasticity and Functional Recovery in Multiple Sclerosis," *Nature Reviews. Neurology* 8, no. 11 (September 18, 2012): 635–46 , https://doi.org/10.1038/nrneurol.2012.179; Marcela Pekna, Milos Pekny, and Michael Nilsson, "Modulation of Neural Plasticity as a Basis for Stroke Rehabilitation," *Stroke* 43, no. 10 (October 2012): 2819–28, https://doi.org/10.1161/strokeaha.112.654228.

24 Luca Colucci-D'Amato and Umberto di Porzio, "Neurogenesis in Adult CNS: from Denial to Opportunities and Challenges for Therapy," *BioEssays* 30, no. 2 (2008): 135–45, https://doi.org/10.1002/bies.20703.

25 E. Taub et al., "The Learned Nonuse Phenomenon: Implications for Rehabilitation," *Europa Medicophysica* 42, no. 3 (September 2006): 241–56, https://pubmed.ncbi. nlm.nih.gov/17039223; J. Liepert et al., "Motor Cortex Plasticity during Constraint-Induced Movement Therapy in Stroke Patients," *Neuroscience Letters,* 250, no. 1 (June 1998): 5–8 https://doi.org/10.1016/s0304-3940(98)00386-3; Edward Taub et al., "An Operant Approach to Rehabilitation Medicine: Overcoming Learned Nonuse by Shaping," *Journal of the Experimental Analysis of Behavior,* 61, no. 2 (March 1994): 281–93, https://doi.org/10.1901/jeab.1994.61-281.

26 Judith D. Schaechter, "Motor Rehabilitation and Brain Plasticity after Hemiparetic Stroke," *Progress in Neurobiology* 73, no. 1 (May 2004): 61–72 , https://doi.org/10.1016/j. pneurobio.2004.04.001; R. J. Nudo et al., "Use-Dependent Alterations of Movement Representations in Primary Motor Cortex of Adult Squirrel Monkeys," *Journal of Neuroscience* 16, no. 2 (January 15, 1996): 785–807, https://doi.org/10.1523/ jneurosci.16-02-00785.1996; Garrett W. Milliken, Erik J. Plautz, and Randolph J. Nudo, "Distal Forelimb Representations in Primary Motor Cortex Are Redistributed after Forelimb Restriction: A Longitudinal Study in Adult Squirrel Monkeys," *Journal of Neurophysiology* 109, no. 5 (March 1, 2013): 1268–82, https://doi.org/10.1152/ jn.00044.2012.

27 K. A. Irvine and W. F. Blakemore, "Remyelination Protects Axons from
    Demyelination-Associated Axon Degeneration," *Brain* 131, no. 6 (January 29, 2008):
    1464–77 https://doi.org/10.1093/brain/awn080; Bjoern Neumann et al. "Remyelination
    and Ageing: Reversing the Ravages of Time," *Multiple Sclerosis Journal* 25, no. 14
    (November 5, 2019): 1835–41, https://doi.org/10.1177/1352458519884006; Verena
    Schultz et al. "Acutely Damaged Axons Are Remyelinated in Multiple Sclerosis
    and Experimental Models of Demyelination," *Glia* 65, no. 8 (May 31, 2017): 1350–60,
    https://doi.org/10.1002/glia.23167; I. D. Duncan et al., "Extensive Remyelination of
    the CNS Leads to Functional Recovery," Proceedings of the *National Academy of
    Sciences* 106, no. 16 (April 2, 2009): 6832–6, https://doi.org/10.1073/pnas.0812500106.

28 R. Pineiro et al., "Functional MRI Detects Posterior Shifts in Primary Sensorimotor
    Cortex Activation After Stroke," *Stroke* 32, no. 5 (May 2001): 1134–9, https://doi.
    org/10.1161/01.str.32.5.1134; Heidi Johansen-Berg et al., "Correlation between Motor
    Improvements and Altered FMRI Activity after Rehabilitative Therapy," *Brain* 125,
    no. 12 (December 2002): 2731–42, https://doi.org/10.1093/brain/awf282; D. Zeller et
    al., "Rapid-Onset Central Motor Plasticity in Multiple Sclerosis," *Neurology* 74, no. 9
    (March 1, 2010): 728–35, https://doi.org/10.1212/wnl.0b013e3181d31dcf.

29 Stefan A. Berghoff et al., "Dietary Cholesterol Promotes Repair of Demyelinated
    Lesions in the Adult Brain," *Nature Communications* 8, no. 1 (January 24, 2017),
    https://doi.org/10.1038/ncomms14241.

30 "The Role of E Stim in Rehab and Recovery: Neurogenerative Diseases or
    Neurological Injuries," *Terry Wahls*, last modified April 17, 2020, https://terrywahls.
    com/role-of-estim-in-rehab-and-recovery-neurodegenerative-diseases-or-
    neurological-injuries.

31 Catherine E. Lang et al., "Observation of Amounts of Movement Practice Provided
    During Stroke Rehabilitation," *Archives of Physical Medicine Rehabilitation* 90, no. 10
    (October 2009): 1692–8, https://doi.org/10.1016/j.apmr.2009.04.005.

32 Norman Doidge, *The Brain that Changes Itself: Stories of Personal Triumph from the
    Frontiers of Brain Science* (New York: Penguin Books, 2007), 90–1.

33 M. M. Merzenich et al., "Progression of Change Following Median Nerve Section in
    the Cortical Representation of the Hand in Areas 3b and 1 in Adult Owl and Squirrel
    Monkeys," *Neuroscience* 10, no. 3 (October 1983): 639–65, https://doi.org/10.1016/0306-
    4522(83)90208-7; J. T. Wall et al., "Functional Reorganization in Somatosensory
    Cortical Areas 3b and 1 of Adult Monkeys after Median Nerve Repair: Possible
    Relationships to Sensory Recovery in Humans," *The Journal of Neuroscience* 6, no. 1
    (January 1, 1986): 218–33, https://doi.org/10.1523/jneurosci.06-01-00218.1986.

34 Guo-li Ming and Hongjun Song, "Adult Neurogenesis in the Mammalian Brain:
    Significant Answers and Significant Questions," *Neuron* 70, no. 4 (May 2011): 687–702,
    https://doi.org/10.1016/j.neuron.2011.05.001.

35 Eric A. Huebner and Stephen M. Strittmatter, "Axon Regeneration in the Peripheral and Central Nervous Systems" in *Results and Problems in Cell Differentiation* (Berlin, Germany: Springer Berlin Heidelberg, 2009), 305–60, https://doi.org/10.1007/400_2009_19; Bart Nieuwenhuis et al., "PI 3-kinase Delta Enhances Axonal PIP 3 to Support Axon Regeneration in the Adult CNS," *EMBO Molecular Medicine* 12, no. 8 (June 17, 2020), https://doi.org/10.15252/emmm.201911674; Zu-Lin Chen, Wei-Ming Yu, and Sidney Strickland, "Peripheral Regeneration," *Annual Review of Neuroscience* 30, no. 1 (July 2007): 209–33, https://doi.org/10.1146/annurev.neuro.30.051606.094337.

36 Sharon A. Gutman, *Neuroscience for Rehabilitation Professionals: The Essential Principles Underlying Rehabilitation Practice*, 3rd ed. {New York: Slack Incorporated,2017), 171.

37 Tessa Gordon, "Electrical Stimulation to Enhance Axon Regeneration After Peripheral Nerve Injuries in Animal Models and Humans," *Neurotherapeutics* 13, no. 2 (January 11, 2016): 295–310, https://doi.org/10.1007/s13311-015-0415-1.

38 K. A. Irvine and W. F. Blakemore, "Remyelination Protects Axons from Demyelination-Associated Axon Degeneration," *Brain* 131, no. 6 (January 29, 2008): 1464–77 https://doi.org/10.1093/brain/awn080; C. Gregg et al., "White Matter Plasticity and Enhanced Remyelination in the Maternal CNS," *Journal of Neuroscience* 27, no. 8 (February 21, 2007): 1812–23, https://doi.org/10.1523/jneurosci.4441-06.2007.

39 Unlike the Neubie, which uses direct current to stimulate and re-educate the muscles and nerves, FES uses alternating current to cause the muscles to contract. Though there can be health benefits to this approach, patients typically develop a reliance on FES machines to do the work.

40 When someone responds quickly to treatment, it's an indicator that they already had that capability inside of them. In other words, neurological stimulation is enabling them to express their existing functional capacity. As I wrote in previous chapters, structural/hardware changes usually take longer to achieve than functional/software changes.

41 V. W. Mark et al., "Constraint-Induced Movement Therapy Can Improve Hemiparetic Progressive Multiple Sclerosis. Preliminary Findings," *Multiple Sclerosis Journal* 14, no. 7 (June 23, 2008): 992–4, https://doi.org/10.1177/1352458508090223; E. Taub et. al., "Technique to Improve Chronic Motor Deficit after Stroke," *Archives of Physical Medicine and Rehabilitation* 74, no. 4 (April 1993):347–54, https://pubmed.ncbi.nlm.nih.gov/8466415; Gitendra Uswatte and Edward Taub, "Constraint-Induced Movement Therapy: A Method for Harnessing Neuroplasticity to Treat Motor Disorders," *Progress in Brain Research* 207 (2013): 379–401, https://doi.org/10.1016/b978-0-444-63327-9.00015-1; Victor W. Mark et al., "Constraint-Induced Movement Therapy for the Lower Extremities in Multiple Sclerosis: Case Series With 4-Year Follow-Up," *Archives of Physical Medicine and Rehabilitation* 94, no. 4 (April 2013): 753–60, https://doi.org/10.1016/j.apmr.2012.09.032.

CHAPTER 6

42 Stephen W. Porges, "Social Engagement and Attachment: A Phylogenetic Perspective," in *The Polyvagal Theory: Neurophysiological Foundations of Emotions, Attachment, Communication, and Self-Regulation* (New York: W.W. Norton & Company, 2011).

43 Robert M. Sapolsky, *Why Zebras Don't Get Ulcers*, 3rd ed. (New York: Holt Paperbacks, 2004).

44 Vladimir M. Zatsiorsky and William J. Kraemer, "Athlete-Specific Strength" in *Science and Practice of Strength Training*, 2nd ed. (Champagne, Illinois: Human Kinetics, 2006); Vladimir M. Zatsiorsky and William J. Kraemer, "Training Intensity" in *Science and Practice of Strength Training*, 2nd ed. (Champagne, Illinois: Human Kinetics, 2006); Pavel Tsatsouline, *Power to the People: Russian Strength Training Secrets for Every American* (Saint Paul, Minnesota: Dragon Door Publications, 1999).

45 Preethi Srikanthan and Arun S. Karlamanga, "Muscle Mass Index as a Predictor of Longevity in Older Adults," *The American Journal of Medicine* 127, no. 6 (June 2014): 547-53, https://doi.org/10.1016/j.amjmed.2014.02.007; S.-Y Chuang et al., "Skeletal Muscle Mass and Risk of Death in an Elderly Population," *Nutrition, Metabolism and Cardiovascular Diseases* 24, no. 7 (July 2014): 784-91, https://doi.org/10.1016/j.numecd.2013.11.010.

46 Rosa Mancinelli et al., "Neuromuscular Electrical Stimulation Induces Skeletal Muscle Fiber Remodeling and Specific Gene Expression Profile in Healthy Elderly," *Frontiers in Physiology* 10 (November 27, 2019), https://doi.org/10.3389/fphys.2019.01459.

47 Eduardo L. Cadore et al., "Multicomponent Exercises Including Muscle Power Training Enhance Muscle Mass, Power Output, and Functional Outcomes in Institutionalized Frail Nonagenarians," *AGE* 36, no. 2 (September 13, 2013): 773-85, https://doi.org/10.1007/s11357-013-9586-z;

48 C. J. Cyron and J. D. Humphrey, "Growth and Remodeling of Load-Bearing Biological Soft Tissues," *Meccanica* 52, no. 3 (June 27, 2016): 645-64, https://doi.org/10.1007/s11012-016-0472-5.

49 P. Vargovic, G. Manz, and R. Kvetnansky, "Continuous Cold Exposure Induces an Anti-Inflammatory Response in Mesenteric Adipose Tissue Associated with Catecholamine Production and Thermogenin Expression in Rats," *Endocrine Regulations* 50, no. 3 (July 1, 2016): 137-44, https://doi.org/10.1515/enr-2016-0015; Gracielle Vieira Ramos et al., "Cryotherapy Reduces Inflammatory Response Without Altering Muscle Regeneration Process and Extracellular Matrix Remodeling of Rat Muscle," *Scientific Reports* 6, no. 1 (January 4, 2016), https://doi.org/10.1038/srep18525; Yizhen Nie et al., "Cold Exposure Stimulates Lipid Metabolism, Induces Inflammatory Response in the Adipose Tissue of Mice and Promotes the Osteogenic Differentiation of BMMSCs via the p38 MAPK Pathway in Vitro," *International Journal of Clinical and Experimental Pathology* 8, no. 9 (September 2015), 10875-86, https://pubmed.ncbi.nlm.nih.gov/26617802.

50   Anouk A. J. J. van der Lans et al. "Cold Acclimation Recruits Human Brown Fat and Increases Nonshivering Thermogenesis," *Journal of Clinical Investigation* 123, no. 8 (July 15, 2013): 3395-3403, https://doi.org/10.1172/jci68993; Wouter van Marken Lichtenbelt et al., "Cold Exposure: an Approach to Increasing Energy Expenditure in Humans," *Trends in Endocrinology & Metabolism* 25, no. 4 (April 2014): 165-7, https://doi.org/10.1016/j.tem.2014.01.001; Véronique Ouellet et al., "Brown Adipose Tissue Oxidative Metabolism Contributes to Energy Expenditure during Acute Cold Exposure in Humans," *Journal of Clinical Investigation* 122, no. 2 (February 1, 2012): 545-52, https://doi.org/10.1172/jci60433.

51   Tiina M. Mäkinen et al., "Autonomic Nervous Function During Whole-Body Cold Exposure Before and After Cold Acclimation," *Aviation, Space, and Environmental Medicine* 79, no. 9 (September 1, 2008): 875-82, https://doi.org/10.3357/asem.2235.2008.

52   Since it's a stressor to the circulatory system, we encourage anyone who wants to experiment with cold exposure to consult a physician first. In addition, we generally encourage people to start slow. Over time, the body will adapt.

53   This discussion of motor units and the associated image are adapted from: Vladimir M. Zatsiorsky and William J. Kraemer, "Training Intensity" in *Science and Practice of Strength Training*, 2nd ed. (Champagne, Illinois: Human Kinetics, 2006); Vladimir M. Zatsiorsky and William J. Kraemer, "Strength Exercises" in *Science and Practice of Strength Training*, 2nd ed. (Champagne, Illinois: Human Kinetics, 2006).

54   Paul C. LaStayo et al., "Eccentric Muscle Contractions: Their Contribution to Injury, Prevention, Rehabilitation, and Sport," *Journal of Orthopaedic & Sports Physical Therapy* 33, no. 10 (October 2003): 557-71, https://doi.org/10.2519/jospt.2003.33.10.557.

55   Frederick Travis et al., "Invincible Athletics Program: Aerobic Exercise and Performance without Strain," *International Journal of Neuroscience* 85, no. 3-4 (January 1996): 301-8, https://doi.org/10.3109/00207459608986691.

56   For a thorough explanation of recovery and adaptation that describes these processes in detail, see: Atko Viru, *Adaptation in Sports Training* (New York: CRC Press, 1995).

57   Martin Gibala, "Molecular Responses to High-Intensity Interval Exercise" *Applied Physiology, Nutrition, and Metabolism* 34, no. 3 (June 2009): 428-32, https://doi.org/10.1139/h09-046; Martin J. Gibala et al., "Physiological Adaptations to Low-Volume, High-Intensity Interval Training in Health and Disease," *The Journal of Physiology* 590, no. 5 (March 1, 2012): 1077-84, https://doi.org/10.1113/jphysiol.2011.224725.

58 Morgan J. Berryman-Maciel et al., "Can Reduced-Exertion, High-Intensity Interval Training Combat the Deleterious Cardiometabolic Effects of a Sedentary Lifestyle?" *International Journal of Research in Exercise Physiology* 14, no. 2 (July 23, 2019): 55–74, https://ijrep.org/can-reduced-exertion-high-intensity-interval-training-combat-the-deleterious-cardiometabolic-effects-of-a-sedentary-lifestyle; Tom Cuddy, Joyce Ramos, and Lance Dalleck, "Reduced Exertion High-Intensity Interval Training Is More Effective at Improving Cardiorespiratory Fitness and Cardiometabolic Health than Traditional Moderate-Intensity Continuous Training," *International Journal of Environmental Research and Public Health* 16, no. 3 (February 7, 2019): 483, https://doi.org/10.3390/ijerph16030483.

CHAPTER 7

59 Michael Yessis, *Build a Better Athlete: What's Wring with American Sports and How to Fix It* (Terre Haute, Indiana: Equilibrium Books, 2006).

60 Vladimir M. Zatsiorsky and William J. Kraemer, "Injury Prevention" in *Science and Practice of Strength Training*, 2nd ed. (Champagne, Illinois: Human Kinetics, 2006).

61 S. N. Blair, "Physical Fitness and All-Cause Mortality. A Prospective Study of Healthy Men and Women," *The Journal of the American Medical Association* 262, no. 17 (November 3, 1989): 2395–2401, https://doi.org/10.1001/jama.262.17.2395; Juliana Antero-Jacquemin et al., "The Heart of the Matter: Years-Saved from Cardiovascular and Cancer Deaths in an Elite Athlete Cohort with over a Century of Follow-Up," *European Journal of Epidemiology* 33, no. 6 (May 5, 2018): 531–43, https://doi.org/10.1007/s10654-018-0401-0; Urho M. Kujala et al., "Associations of Aerobic Fitness and Maximal Muscular Strength With Metabolites in Young Men." *JAMA Network Open* 2, no. 8 (August 23, 2019): e198265, https://doi.org/10.1001/jamanetworkopen.2019.8265.

62 Dona L. Tomlin and Howard A. Wenger, "The Relationship Between Aerobic Fitness and Recovery from High Intensity Intermittent Exercise," *Sports Medicine* 31, no. 1 (2001): 1–11, https://doi.org/10.2165/00007256-200131010-00001.

63 Yuri Verkhoshansky and Natalia Verkhoshansky, *Special Strength Training: Manual for Coaches* (Rome: Verhoshansky.com, 2011), 110–111.

64 Yuri V. Verkhoshansky and Mel c. Siff, *Supertraining*, 6th ed. (Denver, Colorado: Verhoshansky.com, 2009).

65 Kenneth P.Clark, Laurence J. Ryan, and Peter G. Weyand, "A General Relationship Links Gait Mechanics and Running Ground Reaction Forces," *Journal of Experimental Biology* 220, no. 2 (January 1, 2016): 247–58, https://doi.org/10.1242/jeb.138057; Peter G. Weyand et al., "Faster Top Running Speeds Are Achieved with Greater Ground Forces Not More Rapid Leg Movements," *Journal of Applied Physiology* 89, no. 5 (November 1, 2000): 1991–9, https://doi.org/10.1152/jappl.2000.89.5.1991.

66 Two books on plyometrics that I recommend are: Donald Chu, *Jumping into Plyometrics*, 2nd ed. (Champaign, Illinois: Human Kinetics, 1998); James C. Radcliffe and Robert C. Farentinos, *High-Powered Plyometrics* (Champaign, Illinois: Human Kinetics, 1999).

67 Yohei Shimokochi and Sandra J. Shultz, "Mechanisms of Noncontact Anterior Cruciate Ligament Injury," *Journal of Athletic Training* 43, no. 4 (July 1, 2008): 396–408, https://doi.org/10.4085/1062-6050-43.4.396; Eduard Alentorn-Geli et al., "Prevention of Non-Contact Anterior Cruciate Ligament Injuries in Soccer Players. Part 1: Mechanisms of Injury and Underlying Risk Factors," *Knee Surgery, Sports Traumatology, Arthroscopy* 17, no. 7 (May 19, 2009): 705–29, https://doi.org/10.1007/s00167-009-0813-1.

68 Claude Bouchard et al., "Genomic Predictors of the Maximal O2 Uptake Response to Standardized Exercise Training Programs," *Journal of Applied Physiology* 110, no. 5 (May 2011): 1160–70, https://doi.org/10.1152/japplphysiol.00973.2010; C. Lundby, D. Montero, and M. Joyner, "Biology of VO2max: Looking under the Physiology Lamp," *Acta Physiologica* 220, no. 2 (November 25, 2016): 218–28, https://doi.org/10.1111/apha.12827.

69 Yuri Verkhoshansky and Natalia Verkhoshansky, *Special Strength Training: Manual for Coaches* (Rome: Verkhoshansky.com, 2011), XVI.

70 Timothy David Noakes, "Fatigue Is a Brain-Derived Emotion That Regulates the Exercise Behavior to Ensure the Protection of Whole Body Homeostasis," *Frontiers in Physiology* 3 (2012), https://doi.org/10.3389/fphys.2012.00082; T. D. Noakes, J. E. Peltonen, and H. K. Rusko, "Evidence that a Central Governor Regulates Exercise Performance during Acute Hypoxia and Hyperoxia," *Journal of Experimental Biology* 204, no. 18 (Septembere 2001): 3225–34, https://pubmed.ncbi.nlm.nih.gov/11581338.

71 Jonathan D.Witt et al., "Inspiratory Muscle Training Attenuates the Human Respiratory Muscle Metaboreflex," *The Journal of Physiology* 584, no. 3 (October 31, 2007): 1019–28, https://doi.org/10.1113/jphysiol.2007.140855; Juan Lorca-Santiago et al., "Inspiratory Muscle Training in Intermittent Sports Modalities: A Systematic Review," *International Journal of Environmental Research and Public Health* 17, no. 12 (June 21, 2020): 4448, https://doi.org/10.3390/ijerph17124448.

72 Monica J. Hubal et al., "Variability in Muscle Size and Strength Gain after Unilateral Resistance Training," *Medicine & Science in Sports & Exercise* 37, no. 6 (June 2005): 964–72, https://pubmed.ncbi.nlm.nih.gov/15947721; James A. Timmons, "Variability in Training-Induced Skeletal Muscle Adaptation," *Journal of Applied Physiology* 110, no. 3 (March 2011): 846–53, https://doi.org/10.1152/japplphysiol.00934.2010; Øystein Sylta et al., "The Effect of Different High-Intensity Periodization Models on Endurance Adaptations," *Medicine & Science in Sports & Exercise* 48, no. 11 (November 2016): 2165–74, https://doi.org/10.1249/mss.0000000000001007; Theresa N. Mann, Robert P. Lamberts, and Michael I. Lambert, "High Responders and Low Responders: Factors Associated with Individual Variation in Response to Standardized Training," *Sports Medicine* 44, no. 8 (May 8, 2014): 1113–24, https://doi.org/10.1007/s40279-014-0197-3.

73 Knut Sindre Mølmen, Sjur Johansen Øfsteng, and Bent R Rønnesta,. "Block
    Periodization of Endurance Training: A Systematic Review and Meta-Analysis," *Open
    Access Journal of Sports Medicine* 10 (October 2019): 145–60, https://doi.org/10.2147/
    oajsm.s180408; Vladimir B. Issurin, "Benefits and Limitations of Block Periodized
    Training Approaches to Athletes' Preparation: A Review," *Sports Medicine* 46, no. 3
    (November 16, 2015): 329–38, https://doi.org/10.1007/s40279-015-0425-5; Timo Andre
    Bakken, "Effects of Block Periodization Training Versus Traditional Periodization
    Training in Trained Cross Country Skiers" (Grad. Essay 62, The Swedish School of
    Sport and Health Sciences, 2013), http://www.diva-portal.org/smash/get/diva2:689598/
    FULLTEXT01.pdf; Bent R. Rønnestad, Sjur J. Øfsteng, and Stian Ellefsen, "Block
    Periodization of Strength and Endurance Training Is Superior to Traditional
    Periodization in Ice Hockey Players," *Scandinavian Journal of Medicine & Science in
    Sports* 29, no. 2 (November 8, 2018): 180–8, https://doi.org/10.1111/sms.13326.

74 Rich D. Johnston et al., "Effect of Different Repeated-High-Intensity-Effort Bouts
    on Subsequent Running, Skill Performance, and Neuromuscular Function,"
    International Journal of Sports Physiology and Performance 11, no. 3 (April 2016):
    311–8, https://doi.org/10.1123/ijspp.2015-0243; Rich D. Johnston et al., "Influence
    of Physical Contact on Neuromuscular Fatigue and Markers of Muscle Damage
    Following Small-Sided Games," *Journal of Science and Medicine in Sport* 17, no. 5
    (September 2014): 535–40, https://doi.org/10.1016/j.jsams.2013.07.018; Terje Dalen
    and Håvard Lorås, "Monitoring Training and Match Physical Load in Junior Soccer
    Players: Starters versus Substitutes," *Sports* 7, no. 3 (March 19, 2019): 70, https://doi.
    org/10.3390/sports7030070.

75 Callum G. Brownstein et al., "Etiology and Recovery of Neuromuscular Fatigue
    Following Competitive Soccer Match-Play," *Frontiers in Physiology* 8 (October 25,
    2017), https://doi.org/10.3389/fphys.2017.00831; Ermanno Rampinini et al., "Match-
    Related Fatigue in Soccer Players," *Medicine & Science in Sports & Exercise* 43, no. 11
    (November 2011): 2161–70, https://doi.org/10.1249/mss.0b013e31821e9c5c.

CHAPTER 8

76 While heart rate variability measures the interval between heartbeats, respiratory
    sinus arrhythmia (RSA) is the variation in heart rate that occurs during the
    breathing cycle. Since it's directly proportional to heart rate variability, RSA is often
    monitored in tandem with heart rate variability. For the sake of simplicity, I'm using
    heart rate variability as a blanket term that encompasses RSA.

77 There are a number of different formulas we can use to calculate heart rate
    variability (For a great overview, see: Fred Shaffer and J. P. Ginsberg, "An Overview of
    Heart Rate Variability Metrics and Norms," *Frontiers in Public Health* 5 (September
    28, 2017), https://doi.org/10.3389/fpubh.2017.00258.). When measuring heart rate
    variability over time, it's important to use the same formula (i.e., the same device)
    in order to accurately gauge trends and fluctuations. If we compare heart rate
    variability readings using different devices and different formulas, the results can
    be misleading.

78 Stefan Gradl et al., "An Overview of the Feasibility of Permanent, Real-Time, Unobtrusive Stress Measurement with Current Wearables," in *Proceedings of the 13th EAI International Conference on Pervasive Computing Technologies for Healthcare* (New York: Association for Computing Machinery, 2019): 360–5, https://doi.org/10.1145/3329189.3329233; Delaram Jarchi et al., "Estimation of HRV and SpO2 from Wrist-Worn Commercial Sensors for Clinical Settings," in *2018 IEEE 15th International Conference on Wearable and Implantable Body Sensor Networks (BSN)* (New York: IEEE, 2018): 144–7, https://doi.org/10.1109/bsn.2018.8329679; Onur Dur et al., "Design Rationale and Performance Evaluation of the Wavelet Health Wristband: Benchtop Validation of a Wrist-Worn Physiological Signal Recorder," *JMIR MHealth and UHealth* 6, no. 10 (October 16, 2018): e11040, https://doi.org/10.2196/11040; Massimilliano de Zambotti et al., "The Sleep of the Ring: Comparison of the ŌURA Sleep Tracker Against Polysomnography," *Behavioral Sleep Medicine* 17, no. 2 (March 21, 2017): 124–36, https://doi.org/10.1080/15402002.2017.1300587; Hannu Kinnunen, "Sleep Lab Validation of a Wellness Ring in Detecting Sleep Patterns Based on Photoplethysmogram Actigraphy and Body Temperature," *OURA Ring*, last modified February 9, 2016, https://d1aoefioav7lro.cloudfront.net/wp-content/uploads/2018/10/23112923/Validity-of-the-OURA-Ring-in-determining-Sleep-Quantity-and-Quality-2016.pdf.

79 Mitch Leslie, "COVID-19 Fight Enlists Digital Technology: Tracking an Elusive Foe," *Engineering* 6, no. 10 (October 2020): 1061–3, https://doi.org/10.1016/j.eng.2020.08.006.

80 There are many different formulas we can use to calculate estimated maximum heart rate. The 207 − (0.7 × age) formula comes from: Hirofumi Tanaka, Kevin D Monahan, and Douglas R Seals, "Age-Predicted Maximal Heart Rate Revisited," *Journal of the American College of Cardiology* 37, no. 1 (January 2001): 153–6, https://doi.org/10.1016/s0735-1097(00)01054-8.; Yet another alternative formula is this: males = 202 − 0.55 × age and females = 216 − 1.09 × age (G. Whyte et al., "Training Induced Changes in Maximum Heart Rate," *International Journal of Sports Medicine* 29, no. 2 (February 2008): 129–33, https://doi.org/10.1055/s-2007-965783.)

81 Steven Tringali, Charles William Oberer, and Jian Huang, "Low Diastolic Blood Pressure as a Risk for All-Cause Mortality in VA Patients," *International Journal of Hypertension* 2013 (2013): 1–5, https://doi.org/10.1155/2013/178780; Athanase D. Protogerou et al., "Diastolic Blood Pressure and Mortality in the Elderly With Cardiovascular Disease," *Hypertension* 50, no. 1 (July 2007): 172–80, https://doi.org/10.1161/hypertensionaha.107.089797; Grant W. Somes et al., "The Role of Diastolic Blood Pressure When Treating Isolated Systolic Hypertension," *Archives of Internal Medicine* 159, no. 17 (September 27, 1999): 2004, https://doi.org/10.1001/archinte.159.17.2004.

82 Stephen W. Porges, *The Polyvagal Theory: Neurophysiological Foundations of Emotions, Attachment, Communication, and Self-Regulation* (New York: W.W. Norton & Company, 2011).

83 Maarten A.S. Boksem, Theo F. Meijman, and Monicque M. Lorist, "Effects of Mental Fatigue on Attention: An ERP Study," *Cognitive Brain Research* 25, no. 1 (September 2005): 107–16, https://doi.org/10.1016/j.cogbrainres.2005.04.011.

84 Hans Henrik Sievertsen, Francesca Gino, and Marco Piovesan, "Cognitive Fatigue Influences Students' Performance on Standardized Tests," *Proceedings of the National Academy of Sciences* 113, no. 10 (February 16, 2016): 2621–4, https://doi.org/10.1073/pnas.1516947113.

85 O'Dhaniel A.Mullette-Gillman, Ruth L. F. Leong, and Yoanna A. Kurnianingsih, "Cognitive Fatigue Destabilizes Economic Decision Making Preferences and Strategies," *PLoS One* 10, no. 7 (July 31, 2015): e0132022, https://doi.org/10.1371/journal.pone.0132022; G. Robert J. Hockey et al., "Effects of Negative Mood States on Risk in Everyday Decision Making," *Cognition and Emotion* 14, no. 6 (November 2000): 823–55, https://doi.org/10.1080/02699930050156654; Kathleen D. Vohs et al., "Making Choices Impairs Subsequent Self-Control: A Limited-Resource Account of Decision Making, Self-Regulation, and Active Initiative," *Journal of Personality and Social Psychology* 94, no. 5 (May 2008): 883–98, https://doi.org/10.1037/0022-3514.94.5.883.

86 S. Danziger, J. Levav, and L. Avnaim-Pesso, "Extraneous Factors in Judicial Decisions," *Proceedings of the National Academy of Sciences* 108, no. 17 (April 11, 2011): 6889–92, https://doi.org/10.1073/pnas.1018033108.

87 Jeffrey A. Linder et al., "Time of Day and the Decision to Prescribe Antibiotics." *JAMA Internal Medicine* 174, no. 12 (December 1, 2014): 2029, https://doi.org/10.1001/jamainternmed.2014.5225.

88 George Bartzokis et al., "Lifespan Trajectory of Myelin Integrity and Maximum Motor Speed," *Neurobiology of Aging* 31, no. 9 (September 2010): 1554–62, https://doi.org/10.1016/j.neurobiolaging.2008.08.015.

89 Rolf Gruetter, "Glycogen: The Forgotten Cerebral Energy Store," *Journal of Neuroscience Research* 74, no. 2 (October 15, 2003): 179–83, https://doi.org/10.1002/jnr.10785.

90 Nadia Aalling Jessen et al., "The Glymphatic System: A Beginner's Guide," *Neurochemical Research* 40, no. 12 (May 7, 2015): 2583–99, https://doi.org/10.1007/s11064-015-1581-6; Lauren M. Hablitz et al., "Circadian Control of Brain Glymphatic and Lymphatic Fluid Flow," *Nature Communications* 11, no. 1 (September 2, 2020), https://doi.org/10.1038/s41467-020-18115-2; University of Rochester Medical Center, "Not All Sleep is Equal When it Comes to Cleaning the Brain," *Science Daily*, last modified February 27, 2019, www.sciencedaily.com/releases/2019/02/190227173111.htm; Nahid Ahmadian et al., "Review Paper: Tau Pathology of Alzheimer Disease: Possible Role of Sleep Deprivation," *Basic and Clinical Neuroscience Journal* 9, no. 5 (September 30, 2018): 307–16, https://doi.org/10.32598/bcn.9.5.307.

91 A. Karni et al., "Dependence on REM Sleep of Overnight Improvement of a Perceptual Skill," *Science* 265, no. 5172 (July 29, 1994): 679–82, https://doi.org/10.1126/science.8036518; C. T. Smith, "Posttraining Increases in REM Sleep Intensity Implicate REM Sleep in Memory Processing and Provide a Biological Marker of Learning Potential," *Learning & Memory* 11, no. 6 (November 1, 2004): 714–9, https://doi.org/10.1101/lm.74904; Philippe Peigneux et al., "Sleeping Brain, Learning Brain. The Role of Sleep for Memory Systems," *Neuroreport* 12, no. 18 (December 2001): A111–24, https://doi.org/10.1097/00001756-200112210-00001; Werner Plihal and Jan Born, "Effects of Early and Late Nocturnal Sleep on Declarative and Procedural Memory," *Journal of Cognitive Neuroscience* 9, no. 4 (July 1997): 534–47, https://doi.org/10.1162/jocn.1997.9.4.534.

92 Karla A. Kubitz et al., "The Effects of Acute and Chronic Exercise on Sleep," *Sports Medicine* 21, no. 4 (April 1996): 277–91, https://doi.org/10.2165/00007256-199621040-00004; C. Shapiro et al., "Slow-Wave Sleep: A Recovery Period after Exercise," *Science* 214, no. 4526 (December 11, 1981): 1253–4, https://doi.org/10.1126/science.7302594.

93 Institute of Medicine, *Sleep Disorders and Sleep Deprivation: An Unmet Public Health Problem*, eds. Harvey R. Colten and Bruce M. Altevogy (Washington, DC: The National Academies Press, 2006), https://doi.org/10.17226/11617; M. A. Carskadon and W. C. Dement, "Normal Human Sleep: An Overview," in *Principles and Practice of Sleep Medicine* 5th ed.,eds. M. H. Kryger, T. Roth, and W. C. Dement (St. Louis, Missouri: Elsevier Saunders, 2011): 16–26.

94 Massimilliano de Zambotti et al., "The Sleep of the Ring: Comparison of the ŌURA Sleep Tracker Against Polysomnography," *Behavioral Sleep Medicine* 17, no. 2 (March 21, 2017): 124–36, https://doi.org/10.1080/15402002.2017.1300587.

95 Bret H. Goodpaster and Lauren M. Sparks, "Metabolic Flexibility in Health and Disease," *Cell Metabolism* 25, no. 5 (May 2017): 1027–36, https://doi.org/10.1016/j.cmet.2017.04.015.

96 Charikleia Stefanaki et al., "Chronic Stress and Body Composition Disorders: Implications for Health and Disease," *Hormones* 17, no. 1 (March 2018): 33–43, https://doi.org/10.1007/s42000-018-0023-7.

97 This is the American Council on Exercise's percent body fat norms calculator for men and women: https://www.acefitness.org/education-and-resources/lifestyle/tools-calculators/percent-body-fat-calculator. See also: Dympna Gallagher et al., "Healthy Percentage Body Fat Ranges: An Approach for Developing Guidelines Based on Body Mass Index," *The American Journal of Clinical Nutrition* 72, no. 3 (September 1, 2000): 694–701, https://doi.org/10.1093/ajcn/72.3.694.

98 Ran Li et al., "Associations of Muscle Mass and Strength with All-Cause Mortality among US Older Adults," *Medicine & Science in Sports & Exercise* 50, no. 3 (March 2018): 458–67, https://doi.org/10.1249/mss.0000000000001448; Hui Wang et al., "Skeletal Muscle Mass as a Mortality Predictor among Nonagenarians and Centenarians: A Prospective Cohort Study," *Scientific Reports* 9, no. 1 (February 20, 2019), https://doi.org/10.1038/s41598-019-38893-0; E. Jeffrey Metter et al., "Skeletal Muscle Strength as a Predictor of All-Cause Mortality in Healthy Men," *The Journals of Gerontology. Series A, Biological Sciences and Medical Sciences* 57, no. 10 (October 1, 2002): B359–65,. https://doi.org/10.1093/gerona/57.10.b359; Preethi Srikanthan and Arun S. Karlamanga, "Muscle Mass Index as a Predictor of Longevity in Older Adults," *The American Journal of Medicine* 127, no. 6 (June 2014): 547–53, https://doi.org/10.1016/j.amjmed.2014.02.007; Dong Hoon Lee and Edward L Giovannucci, "Body Composition and Mortality in the General Population: A Review of Epidemiologic Studies," *Experimental Biology and Medicine* 243, no. 17–18 (December 2018): 1275–85, https://doi.org/10.1177/1535370218818161.

99 Marilia Carabotti et al., "The Gut-Brain Axis: Interactions Between Enteric Microbiota, Central and Enteric Nervous Systems," *Annals of Gastroenterology* 28, no. 2 (April-June 2015): 203–9, https://pubmed.ncbi.nlm.nih.gov/25830558; Sonia Pellissier et al, "Relationship between Vagal Tone, Cortisol, TNF-Alpha, Epinephrine and Negative Affects in Crohn's Disease and Irritable Bowel Syndrome," *PLoS One* 9, no. 9 (September 10, 2014): e105328, https://doi.org/10.1371/journal.pone.0105328.

100 Gerard Clarke et al., "Minireview: Gut Microbiota: The Neglected Endocrine Organ," *Molecular Endocrinology* 28, no. 8 (August 1, 2014): 1221–38, https://doi.org/10.1210/me.2014-1108; John R.Kelly et al., "Breaking down the Barriers: The Gut Microbiome, Intestinal Permeability and Stress-Related Psychiatric Disorders," *Frontiers in Cellular Neuroscience* 9 (October 14, 2015), https://doi.org/10.3389/fncel.2015.00392; Megan W. Bourassa et al., "Butyrate, Neuroepigenetics and the Gut Microbiome: Can a High Fiber Diet Improve Brain Health?" *Neuroscience Letters* 625 (June 2016): 56–63, https://doi.org/10.1016/j.neulet.2016.02.009; Elizabeth Svoboda, "Could the Gut Microbiome Be Linked to Autism?" *Nature* 577, no. 7792 (January 29, 2020): S14–5, https://doi.org/10.1038/d41586-020-00198-y; Mingyu Xu, "Association Between Gut Microbiota and Autism Spectrum Disorder: A Systematic Review and Meta-Analysis," *Frontiers in Psychiatry* 10 (July 17, 2019), https://doi.org/10.3389/fpsyt.2019.00473; Kelly Servick, "Gut Bacteria May Contribute to Autism Symptoms, Mouse Study Finds." *Science*, May 30, 2019, https://doi.org/10.1126/science.aay2207.

101 Doris Vandeputte et al., "Stool Consistency Is Strongly Associated with Gut Microbiota Richness and Composition, Enterotypes and Bacterial Growth Rates," *Gut* 65, no. 1 (June 11, 2015): 57–62, https://doi.org/10.1136/gutjnl-2015-309618.

102 S. J. Lewis and K. W. Heaton, "Stool Form Scale as a Useful Guide to Intestinal Transit Time," *Scandinavian Journal of Gastroenterology* 32, no. 9 (January 1997): 920–4, https://doi.org/10.3109/00365529709011203.

103 L. P. Degen and S. F. Phillips, "How Well Does Stool Form Reflect Colonic Transit?" *Gut* 39, no. 1 (July 1, 1996): 109–13, https://doi.org/10.1136/gut.39.1.109.

104 Manas Kumar Panigrahi et al., "Defecation Frequency and Stool Form in a Coastal Eastern Indian Population," *Journal of Neurogastroenterology and Motility* 19, no. 3 (July 31, 2013): 374–80, https://doi.org/10.5056/jnm.2013.19.3.374.

105 K. W. Heaton et al., "Defecation Frequency and Timing, and Stool Form in the General Population: A Prospective Study," *Gut* 33, no. 6 (June 1, 1992): 818–24, https://doi.org/10.1136/gut.33.6.818; Gabrio Bassotti, "An Extended Assessment of Bowel Habits in a General Population," *World Journal of Gastroenterology* 10, no. 5 (2004): 713, https://doi.org/10.3748/wjg.v10.i5.713.

106 Suzanne C. Segerstrom and Gregory E. Miller, "Psychological Stress and the Human Immune System: A Meta-Analytic Study of 30 Years of Inquiry," *Psychological Bulletin* 130, no. 4 (2004): 601–30, https://doi.org/10.1037/0033-2909.130.4.601.

107 K. Masuo, "Sympathetic Nerve Hyperactivity Precedes Hyperinsulinemia and Blood Pressure Elevation in a Young, Nonobese Japanese Population," *American Journal of Hypertension* 10, no. 1 (January 1997): 77–83, https://doi.org/10.1016/s0895-7061(96)00303-2; Arnljot Flaa et al., "Increased Sympathetic Reactivity May Predict Insulin Resistance: An 18-Year Follow-up Study," *Metabolism* 57, no. 10 (October 2008): 1422–7, https://doi.org/10.1016/j.metabol.2008.05.012; Mercedes R.Carnethon, "Prospective Investigation of Autonomic Nervous System Function and the Development of Type 2 Diabetes," *Circulation* 107, no. 17 (May 6, 2003): 2190–5, https://doi.org/10.1161/01.cir.0000066324.74807.95; Alicia A. Thorp and Markus P. Schlaich, "Relevance of Sympathetic Nervous System Activation in Obesity and Metabolic Syndrome," *Journal of Diabetes Research* 2015 (2015): 1–11, https://doi.org/10.1155/2015/341583; P. Cavallo Perin, S. Maule, and R. Quadri, "Sympathetic Nervous System, Diabetes, and Hypertension," *Clinical and Experimental Hypertension* 23, no. 1-2 (January 2001): 45–55, https://doi.org/10.1081/ceh-100001196.

108 M. Esler, "The Sympathetic System and Hypertension," *American Journal of Hypertension* 13, no. 6 (June 2000): S99–105, https://doi.org/10.1016/s0895-7061(00)00225-9; Murray Esler and David Kaye, "Sympathetic Nervous System Activation in Essential Hypertension, Cardiac Failure and Psychosomatic Heart Disease," *Journal of Cardiovascular Pharmacology* 35 (2000): S1–7, https://doi.org/10.1097/00005344-200000004-00001.

CHAPTER 9

109 Frederick Travis et al., "Invincible Athletics Program: Aerobic Exercise and Performance without Strain," *International Journal of Neuroscience* 85, no. 3-4 (January 1996): 301–8, https://doi.org/10.3109/00207459608986691.

110 Melvin L. Moss, "The Veloepiglottic Sphincter and Obligate. Nose Breathing in the Neonate," *The Journal of Pediatrics* 67, no. 2 (August 1965): 330–1, https://doi.org/10.1016/s0022-3476(65)80260-8.

111 D. O. Rodenstein et al., "Nasal Occlusion during Sleep in Normal and Near-Miss for Sudden Death Syndrome Infants," *Bulletin Européen de Physiopathologie Respiratoire* 23, no. 3 (May–June 1987), 223–6, https://pubmed.ncbi.nlm.nih.gov/3664013.

112 Benoist Schaal, "Mammary Odor Cues and Pheromones," in *Vitamins & Hormones* (Saint Louis, Missouri: Elsevier, 2010): 83–136, https://doi.org/10.1016/s0083-6729(10)83004-3.

113 Martin Reivich, "Arterial Pco2 and Cerebral Hemodynamics," *American Journal of Physiology-Legacy Content* 206, no. 1 (January 1, 1964): 25–35, https://doi.org/10.1152/ajplegacy.1964.206.1.25; Seymour S. Kety and Carl F. Schmidt, "The Effects of Altered Arterial Tensions of Carbon Dioxide and Oxygen on Cerebral Blood Flow and Cerebral Oxygen Consumption of Normal Young Men," *Journal of Clinical Investigation* 27, no. 4 (July 1, 1948): 484–92, https://doi.org/10.1172/jci101995; A. Battisti-Charbonney, J. Fisher, and J. Duffin, "The Cerebrovascular Response to Carbon Dioxide in Humans," *The Journal of Physiology* 589, no. 12 (June 14, 2011): 3039–48, https://doi.org/10.1113/jphysiol.2011.206052.

114 C. Bohr, K. A. Hasselbach, and A. Krogh, "On the Specific Activity of the Settlements during Respiration," *Acta Physiologica* 16 (1904): 402; William F. Ganong, *Review of Medical Physiology*, 15th ed. (New York: Pearson Professional Education , 1991).

115 J. Huttunen et al., "Effects of Voluntary Hyperventilation on Cortical Sensory Responses," *Experimental Brain Research* 125, no. 3 (March 17, 1999): 248–54, https://doi.org/10.1007/s002210050680; M. Balestrino and G G Somjen, "Concentration of Carbon Dioxide, Interstitial PH and Synaptic Transmission in Hippocampal Formation of the Rat," *The Journal of Physiology* 396, no. 1 (February 1, 1988): 247–66, https://doi.org/10.1113/jphysiol.1988.sp016961.

116 *Medical Physiology: Principles for Clinical Medicine*, 5th ed., eds. Rodney A. Rhoades and David R. Bell (Philadelphia: Wolters Kluwer, 2018).

117 "Breathing Exercise 1: The Control Pause (Part I)," *Buteyko Clinic,* last modified March 19, 2014, https://buteykoclinic.com/breathing-exercise-1-the-control-pause-part-i; See also: N. N. Stanley et al., "Evaluation of Breath Holding in Hypercapnia as a Simple Clinical Test of Respiratory Chemosensitivity," *Thorax* 30, no. 3 (June 1, 1975): 337–43, https://doi.org/10.1136/thx.30.3.337; Maria Barnai et al., "Relationship between Breath-Hold Time and Physical Performance in Patients with Cystic Fibrosis," *European Journal of Applied Physiology* 95, no. 2–3 (July 9, 2005): 172–8, https://doi.org/10.1007/s00421-005-1350-3.

118 Emergency physicians often rely on capnography devices to monitor patient status and determine the severity of their condition. Forward-thinking doctors who understand the importance of carbon dioxide levels also use them. For more information, see: Hamed Aminiahidashti et al., "Applications of End-Tidal Carbon Dioxide (ETCO2) Monitoring in Emergency Department; a Narrative Review," *Emergency* 6, no. 1 (January 15, 2018), https://pubmed.ncbi.nlm.nih.gov/29503830.

119 Sasha Hallett, Fadi Toro, and John V. Ashurst, "Physiology, Tidal Volume," in *StatPearls* (Treasure Island, Florida: StatPearls Publishing; 2020), https://www.ncbi.nlm.nih.gov/books/NBK482502.

120 John B. West, *Respiratory Physiology: The Essentials*, 6th ed. (Philadelphia: Lippincott, Williams and Wilkins, 2000).

121 Roderik J. S. Gerritsen and Guido P. H. Band, "Breath of Life: The Respiratory Vagal Stimulation Model of Contemplative Activity," *Frontiers in Human Neuroscience* 12 (October 9, 2018), https://doi.org/10.3389/fnhum.2018.00397; Bruno Bordoni and Emiliano Zanier, "Anatomic Connections of the Diaphragm Influence of Respiration on the Body System," *Journal of Multidisciplinary Healthcare* 2013 (July 2013), 281–91, https://doi.org/10.2147/jmdh.s45443.

122 Richard L. Young et al., "Sensory and Motor Innervation of the Crural Diaphragm by the Vagus Nerves," *Gastroenterology* 138, no. 3 (March 2010): 1091-1101, https://doi.org/10.1053/j.gastro.2009.08.053.

123 Stefanos Volianitis et al., "Inspiratory Muscle Training Improves Rowing Performance," *Medicine and Science in Sports and Exercise* 33, no. 5 (May 2001): 803-9, https://doi.org/10.1097/00005768-200105000-00020; Makoto Sasaki, Hajime Kurosawa, and Masahiro Kohzuki, "Effects of Inspiratory and Expiratory Muscle Training in Normal Subjects," *Journal of the Japanese Physical Therapy Association* 8, no. 1 (2005): 29-37, https://doi.org/10.1298/jjpta.8.29; Barakat Shahin, "Benefits of Short Inspiratory Muscle Training on Exercise Capacity, Dyspnea, and Inspiratory Fraction in COPD Patients," *International Journal of Chronic Obstructive Pulmonary Disease* 3 (September 2008): 423-7, https://doi.org/10.2147/copd.s1822.

124 Ritu Adhana et al., "The Influence of the 2:1 Yogic Breathing Technique on Essential Hypertension," *Indian Journal of Physiology & Pharmacology* 57, no. 1 (January-March 2013): 38-44, https://pubmed.ncbi.nlm.nih.gov/24020097; R. Viskoper, "Nonpharmacologic Treatment of Resistant Hypertensives by Device-Guided Slow Breathing Exercises," *American Journal of Hypertension* 16, no. 6 (June 2003): 484-7, https://doi.org/10.1016/s0895-7061(03)00571-5; M. H. Schein et al., "Treating Hypertension with a Device That Slows and Regularises Breathing: A Randomised, Double-Blind Controlled Study," *Journal of Human Hypertension* 15, no. 4 (April 2001): 271-8, https://doi.org/10.1038/sj.jhh.1001148; E. Grossman et al., "Breathing-Control Lowers Blood Pressure," *Journal of Human Hypertension* 15, no. 4 (April 2001): 263-9, https://doi.org/10.1038/sj.jhh.1001147; Chacko N. Joseph et al., "Slow Breathing Improves Arterial Baroreflex Sensitivity and Decreases Blood Pressure in Essential Hypertension," *Hypertension* 46, no. 4 (October 2005): 714-8, https://doi.org/10.1161/01.hyp.0000179581.68566.7d.

125 Adrian L. Harris, "Hypoxia—a Key Regulatory Factor in Tumour Growth," *Nature Reviews Cancer* 2, no. 1 (January 2002): 38–47, https://doi.org/10.1038/nrc704; Yonglei Liu et al., "Effect of Chronic Intermittent Hypoxia on Biological Behavior and Hypoxia-Associated Gene Expression in Lung Cancer Cells," *Journal of Cellular Biochemistry* 111, no. 3 (June 21, 2010): 554–63, https://doi.org/10.1002/jcb.22739; I. Almendros et al., "Intermittent Hypoxia Enhances Cancer Progression in a Mouse Model of Sleep Apnoea," *European Respiratory Journal* 39, no. 1 (December 31, 2011): 215–7, https://doi.org/10.1183/09031936.00185110; S. Toffoli and C. Michiels, "Intermittent Hypoxia Is a Key Regulator of Cancer Cell and Endothelial Cell Interplay in Tumours," *FEBS Journal* 275, no. 12 (April 25, 2008): 2991–3002, https://doi.org/10.1111/j.1742-4658.2008.06454.x; Peter Vaupel, "The Role of Hypoxia-Induced Factors in Tumor Progression," *The Oncologist* 9, no. S5 (November 2004): 10–7, https://doi.org/10.1634/theoncologist.9-90005-10; F. Javier Nieto et al., "Sleep-Disordered Breathing and Cancer Mortality," *American Journal of Respiratory and Critical Care Medicine* 186, no. 2 (July 15, 2012): 190–4, https://doi.org/10.1164/rccm.201201-0130OC.

126 Ulf Ekelund et al., "Does Physical Activity Attenuate, or Even Eliminate, the Detrimental Association of Sitting Time with Mortality? A Harmonised Meta-Analysis of Data from More than 1 Million Men and Women," *The Lancet* 388, no. 10051 (September 2016): 1302–10, https://doi.org/10.1016/s0140-6736(16)30370-1.

127 Brooke R. Stephens et al., "Effects of 1 Day of Inactivity on Insulin Action in Healthy Men and Women: Interaction with Energy Intake," *Metabolism* 60, no. 7 (July 2011): 941–9, https://doi.org/10.1016/j.metabol.2010.08.014; Travis J.Saunders et al., "The Acute Metabolic and Vascular Impact of Interrupting Prolonged Sitting: A Systematic Review and Meta-Analysis," *Sports Medicine* 48, no. 10 (August 4, 2018): 2347–66, https://doi.org/10.1007/s40279-018-0963-8; Aviroop Biswas et al., "Sedentary Time and Its Association With Risk for Disease Incidence, Mortality, and Hospitalization in Adults," *Annals of Internal Medicine* 162, no. 2 (January 20, 2015): 123, https://doi.org/10.7326/m14-1651; Ambarish Pandey et al., "Continuous Dose-Response Association Between Sedentary Time and Risk for Cardiovascular Disease," *JAMA Cardiology* 1, no. 5 (August 1, 2016): 575, https://doi.org/10.1001/jamacardio.2016.1567; M. T. Hamilton, D. G. Hamilton, and T. W. Zderic, "Role of Low Energy Expenditure and Sitting in Obesity, Metabolic Syndrome, Type 2 Diabetes, and Cardiovascular Disease," *Diabetes* 56, no. 11 (September 7, 2007): 2655–67, https://doi.org/10.2337/db07-0882.

128 Julia M. Giger et al., "Rapid Muscle Atrophy Response to Unloading: Pretranslational Processes Involving MHC and Actin," *Journal of Applied Physiology* 107, no. 4 (October 2009): 1204–12, https://doi.org/10.1152/japplphysiol.00344.2009; T. W. Buford et al., "Effects of Age and Sedentary Lifestyle on Skeletal Muscle NF- B Signaling in Men," *The Journals of Gerontology. Series A, Biological Sciences and Medical Sciences* 65A, no. 5 (January 2, 2010): 532–7, https://doi.org/10.1093/gerona/glp196; J. Gianoudis, C. A. Bailey, and R. M. Daly, "Associations between Sedentary Behaviour and Body Composition, Muscle Function and Sarcopenia in Community-Dwelling Older Adults," *Osteoporosis International* 26, no. 2 (September 23, 2014): 571–9, https://doi.org/10.1007/s00198-014-2895-y.

129 Geoffrey E. Hespe et al., "Exercise Training Improves Obesity-related Lymphatic Dysfunction," *The Journal of Physiology* 594, no. 15 (April 9, 2016): 4267–82, https://doi.org/10.1113/jp271757.

130 Brendon Burchard, *The Charge: Activating the 10 Human Drives that Make You Feel Alive* (New York: Free Press, 2012): 87.

131 J. A. Levine, "Role of Nonexercise Activity Thermogenesis in Resistance to Fat Gain in Humans," *Science* 283, no. 5399 (January 8, 1999): 212–4, https://doi.org/10.1126/science.283.5399.212; Isaac Debache et al., "Associations of Sensor-Derived Physical Behavior with Metabolic Health: A Compositional Analysis in the Record Multisensor Study," *International Journal of Environmental Research and Public Health* 16, no. 5 (March 1, 2019): 741, https://doi.org/10.3390/ijerph16050741.

132 Sarah L. Arnette and Terry F. Pettijohn, "The Effects of Posture on Self-Perceived Leadership," *International Journal of Business and Social Science* 3, no. 14 (July 2012): 8–13, https://ijbssnet.com/journals/Vol_3_No_14_Special_Issue_July_2012/2.pdf; Pablo Briñol, Richard E. Petty, and Benjamin Wagner, "Body Posture Effects on Self-Evaluation: A Self-Validation Approach," *European Journal of Social Psychology* 39, no. 6 (February 25, 2009): 1053–64, https://doi.org/10.1002/ejsp.607; Dana R. Carney, Amy J.C. Cuddy, and Andy J. Yap, "Power Posing," *Psychological Science* 21, no. 10 (September 20, 2010): 1363–8, https://doi.org/10.1177/0956797610383437; Amy J. C. Cuddy et al., "Preparatory Power Posing Affects Nonverbal Presence and Job Interview Performance," *Journal of Applied Psychology* 100, no. 4 (July 2015): 1286–95, https://doi.org/10.1037/a0038543; Li Huang et al., "Powerful Postures Versus Powerful Roles," *Psychological Science* 22, no. 1 (December 13, 2010): 95–102, https://doi.org/10.1177/0956797610391912; Erik Peper et al., "Increase Strength and Mood with Posture," *Biofeedback* 44, no. 2 (June 1, 2016): 66–72, https://doi.org/10.5298/1081-5937-44.2.04.

133 Tatiana El Bacha et al., "Dynamic Adaptation of Nutrient Utilization in Humans," *Nature Education* 3, no. 9 (2010): 8, https://www.nature.com/scitable/topicpage/dynamic-adaptation-of-nutrient-utilization-in-humans-14232807.

134 Jeff S. Volek, "Testosterone and Cortisol in Relationship to Dietary Nutrients and Resistance Exercise," *Journal of Applied Physiology* 82, no. 1 (January 1, 1997): 49–54, https://doi.org/10.1152/jappl.1997.82.1.49; M. J. Reed et al., "Dietary Lipids : An Additional Regulator of Plasma Levels of Sex Hormone Binding Globulin," *The Journal of Clinical Endocrinology & Metabolism* 64, no. 5 (May 1987): 1083–5, https://doi.org/10.1210/jcem-64-5-1083.

135 Stefan A. Berghoff et al., "Dietary Cholesterol Promotes Repair of Demyelinated Lesions in the Adult Brain," *Nature Communications* 8, no. 1 (January 24, 2017), https://doi.org/10.1038/ncomms14241.

136 L. Dupuis et al., "Dyslipidemia Is a Protective Factor in Amyotrophic Lateral Sclerosis," *Neurology* 70, no. 13 (January 16, 2008): 1004–9, https://doi.org/10.1212/01.wnl.0000285080.70324.27.

137 M. M. Mielke et al., "High Total Cholesterol Levels in Late Life Associated with a Reduced Risk of Dementia," *Neurology* 64, no. 10 (April 20, 2005): 1689–95, https://doi.org/10.1212/01.wnl.0000161870.78572.a5.

138 L. L. Smith et al., "The Impact of a Repeated Bout of Eccentric Exercise on Muscular Strength, Muscle Soreness and Creatine Kinase," *British Journal of Sports Medicine* 28, no. 4 (December 1, 1994): 267–71, https://doi.org/10.1136/bjsm.28.4.267; Steven E. Riechman et al., "Dietary Cholesterol and Skeletal Muscle Hypertrophy with Resistance Training: A Randomized Placebo-Controlled Trial," *The FASEB Journal* 22, no. S1 (March 1, 2008): 962.13, https://faseb.onlinelibrary.wiley.com/doi/abs/10.1096/fasebj.22.1_supplement.962.13; S. E. Riechman et al., "Statins and Dietary and Serum Cholesterol Are Associated With Increased Lean Mass Following Resistance Training," *The Journals of Gerontology. Series A, Biological Sciences and Medical Sciences* 62, no. 10 (October 1, 2007): 1164–71, https://doi.org/10.1093/gerona/62.10.1164.

139 Stephanie L. Di Stasi et al., "Effects of Statins on Skeletal Muscle: A Perspective for Physical Therapists," *Physical Therapy* 90, no. 10 (October 1, 2010): 1530–42, https://doi.org/10.2522/ptj.20090251; Irfan Esenkaya and Koray Unay, "Tendon, Tendon Healing, Hyperlipidemia and Statins," *Muscles, Ligaments and Tendons Journal* 1, no. 4 (April 1, 2012): 169–71, https://pubmed.ncbi.nlm.nih.gov/23738266; Catherine Buettner et al., "Prevalence of Musculoskeletal Pain and Statin Use," *Journal of General Internal Medicine* 23, no. 8 (May 1, 2008): 1182–6, https://doi.org/10.1007/s11606-008-0636-7; Sofia G. Tsouli et al., "Regression of Achilles Tendon Thickness after Statin Treatment in Patients with Familial Hypercholesterolemia: An Ultrasonographic Study," *Atherosclerosis* 205, no. 1 (July 2009): 151–5, https://doi.org/10.1016/j.atherosclerosis.2008.10.032; Raja C. Pullatt et al., "Tendon Rupture Associated With Simvastatin/Ezetimibe Therapy," *The American Journal of Cardiology* 100, no. 1 (July 2007): 152–3, https://doi.org/10.1016/j.amjcard.2007.02.068; Oludamilola W. Oluleye et al., "Association Between Statin Use and Sex Hormone in the Multi-Ethnic Study of Atherosclerosis Cohort," *The Journal of Clinical Endocrinology & Metabolism* 104, no. 10 (June 3, 2019): 4600–6, https://doi.org/10.1210/jc.2019-00530.

140 Aldons J. Lusis, "Atherosclerosis," *Nature* 407, no. 6801 (September 2000): 233–41, https://doi.org/10.1038/35025203; D. D. Adams, "The Great Cholesterol Myth; Unfortunate Consequences of Brown and Goldstein's Mistake," *QJM* 104, no. 10 (June 20, 2011): 867–70, https://doi.org/10.1093/qjmed/hcr087; G. Taubes, "Cardiovascular Disease: Does Inflammation Cut to the Heart of the Matter?" *Science* 296, no. 5566 (April 12, 2002): 242–5, https://doi.org/10.1126/science.296.5566.242; Andrew Mente et al., "A Systematic Review of the Evidence Supporting a Causal Link Between Dietary Factors and Coronary Heart Disease," *Archives of Internal Medicine* 169, no. 7 (April 13, 2009): 659, https://doi.org/10.1001/archinternmed.2009.38; Rajiv Chowdhury et al., "Association of Dietary, Circulating, and Supplement Fatty Acids with Coronary Risk: A Systematic Review and Meta-Analysis,"*Annals of Internal Medicine* 160, no. 6 (March 18, 2014): 398–406, https://doi.org/10.7326/m13-1788.

141 Robert M. Sapolsky, *Why Zebras Don't Get Ulcers*, 3rd ed. (New York: Holt Paperbacks, 2004).

142 Brittanie M. Volk et al., "Effects of Step-Wise Increases in Dietary Carbohydrate on Circulating Saturated Fatty Acids and Palmitoleic Acid in Adults with Metabolic Syndrome," PLoS One 9, no. 11 (November 21, 2014): e113605, https://doi.org/10.1371/journal.pone.0113605.

143 This article from the *Journal of the American Medical Association* describes how some of the early research blaming fat for the prevalence of heart disease became accepted in part because of the sugar industry, which wanted to downplay evidence about the dangers of sugar among the public and the scientific community: Cristin E. Kearns, Laura A. Schmidt, and Stanton A. Glantz, "Sugar Industry and Coronary Heart Disease Research," *JAMA Internal Medicine* 176, no. 11 (November 1, 2016): 1680, https://doi.org/10.1001/jamainternmed.2016.5394.

144 Christopher E. Ramsden et al., "N-6 Fatty Acid-Specific and Mixed Polyunsaturate Dietary Interventions Have Different Effects on CHD Risk: A Meta-Analysis of Randomised Controlled Trials," *British Journal of Nutrition* 104, no. 11 (December 1, 2010): 1586–1600, https://doi.org/10.1017/s0007114510004010; Christopher E. Ramsden et al., "Re-Evaluation of the Traditional Diet-Heart Hypothesis: Analysis of Recovered Data from Minnesota Coronary Experiment (1968-73)," *BMJ* 353 (April 12, 2016), https://doi.org/10.1136/bmj.i1246; Rajiv Chowdhury et al., "Association of Dietary, Circulating, and Supplement Fatty Acids with Coronary Risk: A Systematic Review and Meta-Analysis,"*Annals of Internal Medicine* 160, no. 6 (March 18, 2014): 398–406, https://doi.org/10.7326/m13-1788; Steven Hamley, "The Effect of Replacing Saturated Fat with Mostly N-6 Polyunsaturated Fat on Coronary Heart Disease: A Meta-Analysis of Randomised Controlled Trials," *Nutrition Journal* 16, no. 1 (May 19, 2017), https://doi.org/10.1186/s12937-017-0254-5.

145 Matthew W. Gillman et al., "Margarine Intake and Subsequent Coronary Heart Disease in Men," *Epidemiology* 8, no. 2 (March 1997): 144–9, https://doi.org/10.1097/00001648-199703000-00004; Robert Clarke and Sarah Lewington, "Trans Fatty Acids and Coronary Heart Disease," *BMJ* 333, no. 7561 (July 27, 2006): 214, https://doi.org/10.1136/bmj.333.7561.214 Qi Sun et al., "A Prospective Study of Trans Fatty Acids in Erythrocytes and Risk of Coronary Heart Disease," *Circulation* 115, no. 14 (April 10, 2007): 1858–65, https://doi.org/10.1161/circulationaha.106.679985; Claudia M. Oomen et al., "Association between Trans Fatty Acid Intake and 10-Year Risk of Coronary Heart Disease in the Zutphen Elderly Study: A Prospective Population-Based Study," *The Lancet* 357, no. 9258 (March 2001): 746–51, https://doi.org/10.1016/s0140-6736(00)04166-0; Michael Lefevre et al., "Comparison of the Acute Response to Meals Enriched with Cis- or Trans-Fatty Acids on Glucose and Lipids in Overweight Individuals with Differing FABP2 Genotypes," *Metabolism* 54, no. 12 (December 2005): 1652–8, https://doi.org/10.1016/j.metabol.2005.06.015; Ahamed Ibrahim, Saravanan Natarajan, and Ghafoorunissa, "Dietary Trans–Fatty Acids Alter Adipocyte Plasma Membrane Fatty Acid Composition and Insulin Sensitivity in Rats," *Metabolism* 54, no. 2 (February 2005): 240–6, https://doi.org/10.1016/j.metabol.2004.08.019; Kylie Kavanagh et al., "Trans Fat Diet Induces Abdominal Obesity and Changes in Insulin Sensitivity in Monkeys," *Obesity* 15, no. 7 (July 2007): 1675–84, https://doi.org/10.1038/oby.2007.200; Dariush Mozaffarian et al., "Dietary Intake of Trans Fatty Acids and Systemic Inflammation in Women," *The American Journal of Clinical Nutrition* 79, no. 4 (April 1, 2004): 606–12, https://doi.org/10.1093/ajcn/79.4.606.

146 When considering dietary changes, food sensitivity testing can be worthwhile, particularly for people with digestive issues. Many functional medicine doctors perform food sensitivity tests, and there also are a variety of viable at-home testing options, including Everlywell and Viome (for more information, see Appendix 2).

147 Mark Sisson, *The Primal Blueprint* (Malibu, California: Primal Nutrition, Inc., 2012).

148 Mehrdad Alirezaei et al., "Short-Term Fasting Induces Profound Neuronal Autophagy," *Autophagy* 6, no. 6 (August 16, 2010): 702–10, https://doi.org/10.4161/auto.6.6.12376.

149 James B. Johnson et al., "Alternate Day Calorie Restriction Improves Clinical Findings and Reduces Markers of Oxidative Stress and Inflammation in Overweight Adults with Moderate Asthma," *Free Radical Biology and Medicine* 42, no. 5 (March 2007): 665–74, https://doi.org/10.1016/j.freeradbiomed.2006.12.005; Fehime B. Aksungar, Aynur E. Topkaya, and Mahmut Akyildiz, "Interleukin-6, C-Reactive Protein and Biochemical Parameters during Prolonged Intermittent Fasting," *Annals of Nutrition and Metabolism* 51, no. 1 (2007): 88–95, https://doi.org/10.1159/000100954.

150 Veerendra Kumar Madala Halagappa et al., "Intermittent Fasting and Caloric Restriction Ameliorate Age-Related Behavioral Deficits in the Triple-Transgenic Mouse Model of Alzheimer's Disease," *Neurobiology of Disease* 26, no. 1 (April 2007): 212–20, https://doi.org/10.1016/j.nbd.2006.12.019; Dale E. Bredesen, "Reversal of Cognitive Decline: A Novel Therapeutic Program," *Aging* 6, no. 9 (September 27, 2014): 707–17, https://doi.org/10.18632/aging.100690; Bronwen Martin, Mark P. Mattson, and Stuart Maudsley, "Caloric Restriction and Intermittent Fasting: Two Potential Diets for Successful Brain Aging." Ageing Research Reviews 5, no. 3 (August 2006): 332–53. https://doi.org/10.1016/j.arr.2006.04.002.

151 Israel Siegel, "Effects of Short-Term Dietary Restriction on Survival of Mammary Ascites Tumor-Bearing Rats," *Cancer Investigation* 6, no. 6 (January 1988): 677–80, https://doi.org/10.3109/07357908809078034; C. Lee et al., "Fasting Cycles Retard Growth of Tumors and Sensitize a Range of Cancer Cell Types to Chemotherapy," *Science Translational Medicine* 4, no. 124 (February 8, 2012): 124ra27-124ra27, https://doi.org/10.1126/scitranslmed.3003293; Olivier Descamps, "Mitochondrial Production of Reactive Oxygen Species and Incidence of Age-Associated Lymphoma in OF1 Mice: Effect of Alternate-Day Fasting," *Mechanisms of Ageing and Development* 126, no. 11 (November 2005): 1185–91, https://doi.org/10.1016/j.mad.2005.06.007; Noeme Sousa Rocha et al., "Effects of Fasting and Intermittent Fasting on Rat Hepatocarcinogenesis Induced by Diethylnitrosamine," *Teratogenesis, Carcinogenesis, and Mutagenesis* 22, no. 2 (2002): 129–38, https://doi.org/10.1002/tcm.10005.

152 Krista A. Varady et al., "Short-Term Modified Alternate-Day Fasting: A Novel Dietary Strategy for Weight Loss and Cardioprotection in Obese Adults," *The American Journal of Clinical Nutrition* 90, no. 5 (September 30, 2009): 1138–43, https://doi.org/10.3945/ajcn.2009.28380; Fernanda Reis de Azevedo, Dimas Ikeoka, and Bruno Caramelli, "Effects of Intermittent Fasting on Metabolism in Men," *Revista Da Associação Médica Brasileira* 59, no. 2 (March 2013): 167–73, https://doi.org/10.1016/j.ramb.2012.09.003; Rona Antoni et al., "The Effects of Intermittent Energy Restriction on Indices of Cardiometabolic Health," *Research in Endocrinology*, June 28, 2014, 1–24, https://doi.org/10.5171/2014.459119.

153 Leonie K. Heilbronn et al., "Alternate-Day Fasting in Nonobese Subjects: Effects on Body Weight, Body Composition, and Energy Metabolism," *The American Journal of Clinical Nutrition* 81, no. 1 (January 1, 2005): 69–73, https://doi.org/10.1093/ajcn/81.1.69; Adrienne R. Barnosky et al., "Intermittent Fasting vs Daily Calorie Restriction for Type 2 Diabetes Prevention: A Review of Human Findings," *Translational Research* 164, no. 4 (October 2014): 302–11, https://doi.org/10.1016/j.trsl.2014.05.013.

154 Donald R. Davis, Melvin D. Epp, and Hugh D. Riordan, "Changes in USDA Food Composition Data for 43 Garden Crops, 1950 to 1999," *Journal of the American College of Nutrition* 23, no. 6 (December 2004): 669–82, https://doi.org/10.1080/07315724.2004.10719409.

155 "Minerals," MedlinePlus, accessed February 7, 2021, https://medlineplus.gov/minerals.html.

156 Małgorzata Wrzosek et al., "Vitamin D and the Central Nervous System," *Pharmacological Reports* 65, no. 2 (March 2013): 271–8, https://doi.org/10.1016/s1734-1140(13)71003-x; T. Holmøy and S. M. Moen, "Assessing Vitamin D in the Central Nervous System," *Acta Neurologica Scandinavica* 122 (July 2010): 88–92, https://doi.org/10.1111/j.1600-0404.2010.01383.x.

157 David Kennedy, "B Vitamins and the Brain: Mechanisms, Dose and Efficacy—A Review," *Nutrients* 8, no. 2 (January 27, 2016): 68, https://doi.org/10.3390/nu8020068.

158 Calliandra B. Harris et al., "Dietary Pyrroloquinoline Quinone (PQQ) Alters Indicators of Inflammation and Mitochondrial-Related Metabolism in Human Subjects," *The Journal of Nutritional Biochemistry* 24, no. 12 (December 2013): 2076–84, https://doi.org/10.1016/j.jnutbio.2013.07.008; R. T. Matthews et al., "Coenzyme Q10 Administration Increases Brain Mitochondrial Concentrations and Exerts Neuroprotective Effects," *Proceedings of the National Academy of Sciences* 95, no. 15 (July 21, 1998): 8892–7, https://doi.org/10.1073/pnas.95.15.8892.

159 Michael Boschmann et al., "Water-Induced Thermogenesis," *The Journal of Clinical Endocrinology & Metabolism* 88, no. 12 (December 1, 2003): 6015–9, https://doi.org/10.1210/jc.2003-030780.

160 Carl V. Gisolfi, "Water Requirements During Exercise in the Heat," in *Nutritional Needs in Hot Environments: Applications for Military Personnel in Field Operations*, ed. Bernadette M. Marriott (Washington, DC: National Academies Press, 1993): 87–96, https://doi.org/10.17226/2094.

161 Zohreh Kheradpisheh et al., "Impact of Drinking Water Fluoride on Human Thyroid Hormones: A Case- Control Study," *Scientific Reports* 8, no. 1 (February 8, 2018), https://doi.org/10.1038/s41598-018-20696-4; Ashley J. Malin et al., "Fluoride Exposure and Thyroid Function among Adults Living in Canada: Effect Modification by Iodine Status," *Environment International* 121 (December 2018): 667–74, https://doi.org/10.1016/j.envint.2018.09.026.

162 R. D. Morris, "Drinking Water and Cancer," *Environmental Health Perspectives* 103, no. suppl 8 (November 1995): 225–31, https://doi.org/10.1289/ehp.95103s8225.

163 Duck H. Suh, Mohamed S. Abdel-Rahman, and Richard J. Bull, "Effect of Chlorine Dioxide and Its Metabolites in Drinking Water on Fetal Development in Rats," *Journal of Applied Toxicology* 3, no. 2 (April 1983): 75–9, https://doi.org/10.1002/jat.2550030204; Bing-Fang Hwang, Jouni JK Jaakkola, and How-Ran Guo, "Water Disinfection By-Products and the Risk of Specific Birth Defects: A Population-Based Cross-Sectional Study in Taiwan," *Environmental Health* 7, no. 1 (June 2, 2008), https://doi.org/10.1186/1476-069x-7-23.

164 Elina Jerschow et al., "Dichlorophenol-Containing Pesticides and Allergies: Results from the US National Health and Nutrition Examination Survey 2005-2006," *Annals of Allergy, Asthma & Immunology* 109, no. 6 (December 2012): 420–5, https://doi.org/10.1016/j.anai.2012.09.005.

165 There are times when training in a fasted state has health benefits. For people practicing intermittent fasting, it can help promote metabolic flexibility. Along these lines, some bodybuilders have success with an approach known as "fasted cardio." The idea behind fasted cardio is that doing cardio work in a fasted state burns body fat stores. However, this strategy is a minor component of some professional bodybuilders' training regimens, and we don't generally recommend it when we're concerned about high performance within the session. See: Corby K. Martin et al., "Effect of Calorie Restriction on Resting Metabolic Rate and Spontaneous Physical Activity," *Obesity* 15, no. 12 (December 2007): 2964–73, https://doi.org/10.1038/oby.2007.354; Leanne M. Redman et al., "Metabolic and Behavioral Compensations in Response to Caloric Restriction: Implications for the Maintenance of Weight Loss," *PLoS One* 4, no. 2 (February 9, 2009): e4377, https://doi.org/10.1371/journal.pone.0004377.

166 R. H. Goo et al., "Circadian Variation in Gastric Emptying of Meals in Humans," *Gastroenterology* 93, no. 3 (September 1987): 515–8, https://doi.org/10.1016/0016-5085(87)90913-9.

167 C. Czeisler et al., "Human Sleep: Its Duration and Organization Depend on Its Circadian Phase," *Science* 210, no. 4475 (December 12, 1980): 1264–7, https://doi.org/10.1126/science.7434029.

168 Raffaello Furlan et al., "Modifications of Cardiac Autonomic Profile Associated With a Shift Schedule of Work," *Circulation* 102, no. 16 (October 17, 2000): 1912–6, https://doi.org/10.1161/01.cir.102.16.1912.

169 Benjamin L. Smarr et al., "A Time to Remember: The Role of Circadian Clocks in Learning and Memory," *Behavioral Neuroscience* 128, no. 3 (2014): 283–303, https://doi.org/10.1037/a0035963; Kenneth P. Wright, Jr. et al., "Sleep and Wakefulness Out of Phase with Internal Biological Time Impairs Learning in Humans," *Journal of Cognitive Neuroscience* 18, no. 4 (April 1, 2006): 508–21, https://doi.org/10.1162/jocn.2006.18.4.508.

170 David C. Holzman, "What's in a Color? The Unique Human Health Effects of Blue Light," *Environmental Health Perspectives* 118, no. 1 (January 2010), https://doi.org/10.1289/ehp.118-a22; Jeanne F. Duffy and Charles A. Czeisler, "Effect of Light on Human Circadian Physiology," *Sleep Medicine Clinics* 4, no. 2 (June 2009): 165–77, https://doi.org/10.1016/j.jsmc.2009.01.004.

171 Joshua J. Gooley et al., "Exposure to Room Light before Bedtime Suppresses Melatonin Onset and Shortens Melatonin Duration in Humans," *The Journal of Clinical Endocrinology & Metabolism* 96, no. 3 (March 1, 2011): E463–72, https://doi.org/10.1210/jc.2010-2098; Mariana G. Figueiro et al., "The Impact of Light from Computer Monitors on Melatonin Levels in College Students," *Neuroendocrinology Letters* 32, no. 2 (2011): 158–63, https://pubmed.ncbi.nlm.nih.gov/21552190; Russel J. Reiter et al., "Obesity and Metabolic Syndrome: Association with Chronodisruption, Sleep Deprivation, and Melatonin Suppression," *Annals of Medicine* 44, no. 6 (September 2012): 564–77, https://doi.org/10.3109/07853890.2011.586365; Alberto Dominguez-Rodriguez et al., "Melatonin and Circadian Biology in Human Cardiovascular Disease," *Journal of Pineal Research* 49, no. 1 (May 2010): 14–22, https://doi.org/10.1111/j.1600-079x.2010.00773.x; M. A. Quera Salva et al., "Circadian Rhythms, Melatonin and Depression," *Current Pharmaceutical Design* 17, no. 15 (May 1, 2011): 1459–70, https://doi.org/10.2174/138161211796197188; Scott Davis and Dana K. Mirick, "Circadian Disruption, Shift Work and the Risk of Cancer: A Summary of the Evidence and Studies in Seattle," *Cancer Causes & Control* 17, no. 4 (May 2006): 539–45, https://doi.org/10.1007/s10552-005-9010-9.

172 Brittany Wood, "Light Level and Duration of Exposure Determine the Impact of Self-Luminous Tablets on Melatonin Suppression," *Applied Ergonomics* 44, no. 2 (March 2013): 237–40, https://doi.org/10.1016/j.apergo.2012.07.008; Alexandre Sasseville, "Blue Blocker Glasses Impede the Capacity of Bright Light to Suppress Melatonin Production," *Journal of Pineal Research* 41, no. 1 (August 2006): 73–8, https://doi.org/10.1111/j.1600-079x.2006.00332.x; Kimberly Burkhart and James R. Phelps "Amber Lenses to Block Blue Light and Improve Sleep: A Randomized Trial," *Chronobiology International* 26, no. 8 (December 2009): 1602–12, https://doi.org/10.3109/07420520903523719.

173 Edward C. Harding, Nicholas P Franks, and William Wisden, "Sleep and Thermoregulation," *Current Opinion in Physiology* 15 (June 2020): 7–13, https://doi.org/10.1016/j.cophys.2019.11.008.

174 Y. Kutsenko, *Tribuna Masterov* (1963), translated by Andrew Charniga, Jr. (Sportivny Press).

175 M. Giacomoni, F. Billaut, and G. Falgairette, "Effects of the Time of Day on Repeated
All-Out Cycle Performance and Short-Term Recovery Patterns," *International Journal
of Sports Medicine* 27, no. 6 (June 2006): 468–74, https://doi.org/10.1055/s-2005-865822;
V. I. Shaposhnikova, "The Biological Clock," as translated in M. Yessis, *Review of
Soviet Physical Education and Sports* 6, no. 1 (March 1971); A. Nicolas et al., "Time-
of-Day Effects on Myoelectric and Mechanical Properties of Muscle During Maximal
and Prolonged Isokinetic Exercise," *Chronobiology International* 22, no. 6 (January
2005): 997–1011, https://doi.org/10.1080/07420520500397892.

APPENDIX 1

176 Yihong Chen et al., "Physiological Electric Field Works via the VEGF Receptor to
Stimulate Neovessel Formation of Vascular Endothelial Cells in a 3D Environment,"
Biology Open 7, no. 9 (September 15, 2018), https://doi.org/10.1242/bio.035204; Wei-
Wen Hu et al., "The Effects of Substrate-mediated Electrical Stimulation on the
Promotion of Osteogenic Differentiation and Its Optimization," *Journal of Biomedical
Materials Research Part B Applied Biomaterials* 107, no. 5 (October 14, 2018): 1607–19,
https://doi.org/10.1002/jbm.b.34253; Mahmoud Rouabhia et al., "Electrical Stimulation
Promotes Wound Healing by Enhancing Dermal Fibroblast Activity and Promoting
Myofibroblast Transdifferentiation," *PLoS One* 8, no. 8 (August 19, 2013), https://
doi.org/10.1371/journal.pone.0071660; R. B. Borgens, J. W. Vanable, and L. F. Jaffe,
"Bioelectricity and Regeneration. I. Initiation of Frog Limb Regeneration by Minute
Currents," *Journal of Experimental Zoology* 200, no. 3 (June 1977): 403–16, https://
doi.org/10.1002/jez.1402000310; Liudmila P. Leppik et al., "Effects of Electrical
Stimulation on Rat Limb Regeneration, a New Look at an Old Model," *Scientific
Reports* 5, no. 1 (December 17, 2015), https://doi.org/10.1038/srep18353; Colin D.
McCaig et al., "Controlling Cell Behavior Electrically: Current Views and Future
Potential," *Physiological Reviews* 85, no. 3 (July 2005): 943–78, https://doi.org/10.1152/
physrev.00020.2004.

APPENDIX 2

177 Emeran A. Mayer, Kirsten Tillisch, and Arpana Gupta, "Gut/Brain Axis and the
Microbiota," *Journal of Clinical Investigation* 125, no. 3 (February 17, 2015): 926–38,
https://doi.org/10.1172/jci76304; Mona Dehhaghi, Hamed Kazemi Shariat Panahi, and
Gilles J. Guillemin, "Microorganisms' Footprint in Neurodegenerative Diseases,"
Frontiers in Cellular Neuroscience 12 (December 4, 2018), https://doi.org/10.3389/
fncel.2018.00466; Rachel D. Moloney et al., "The Microbiome: Stress, Health and
Disease," *Mammalian Genome* 25, no. 1–2 (November 27, 2013): 49–74, https://doi.
org/10.1007/s00335-013-9488-5.